THE RESILIENT MENTAL HEALTH PRACTICE

The Resilient Mental Health Practice: Nourishing Your Business, Your Clients, and Yourself is a fundamental resource for mental health professionals, designed to serve as a comprehensive yet parsimonious handbook to inspire and inform novice, developing, and experienced mental health professionals. Replete with case studies, *The Resilient Mental Health Practice* gives readers a big-picture view of private practice, including detailed explorations of various topics related to therapist self-care and preventing burnout. Chapters provide a range of ways in which clinicians can build a resilient and sustainable practice while also taking care of their clients and themselves.

Jennifer M. Ossege, PsyD, is the cofounder and managing partner of Viewpoint Psychological Services, PLLC, a group private practice in the Northern Kentucky/Cincinnati area. She is a faculty member and associate director of clinical training in the PsyD program in clinical psychology at Union Institute & University, and she is an adjunct faculty member in the psychology department at Xavier University in Cincinnati. Her website is www.viewpointpsych.com.

Richard W. Sears, PsyD, PhD, MBA, ABPP, is a board-certified clinical psychologist, consultant, and speaker in private practice in Cincinnati and is the director of the Center for Clinical Mindfulness & Meditation. He is also a clinical/research faculty member at the University of Cincinnati Center for Integrative Health and Wellness, volunteer associate professor of psychiatry and behavioral neurosciences at University of Cincinnati College of Medicine, and clinical assistant professor at Wright State University School of Professional Psychology. Dr. Sears is author of ten books on mindfulness, CBT, spirituality, and organizational consultation. His website is www.psych-insights.com.

THE RESILIENT MENTAL HEALTH PRACTICE

NOURISHING YOUR BUSINESS, YOUR CLIENTS, AND YOURSELF

Edited by
Jennifer M. Ossege and
Richard W. Sears

Routledge
Taylor & Francis Group
NEW YORK AND LONDON

First published 2017
by Routledge
605 Third Avenue, New York, NY 10017

and by Routledge
2 Park Square, Milton Park, Abingdon, Oxon, OX14 4RN

Routledge is an imprint of the Taylor & Francis Group, an informa business

Library of Congress Cataloging-in-Publication Data
Names: Ossege, Jennifer M., editor. | Sears, Richard W., 1969– editor.
Title: The resilient mental health practice: nourishing your business, your clients, and yourself / edited by Jennifer M. Ossege and Richard W. Sears.
Description: New York, NY: Routledge, 2017. | Includes bibliographical references and index.
Identifiers: LCCN 2016017679 | ISBN 9781138935884 (hardback: alk. paper) | ISBN 9781138935891 (pbk.: alk. paper) | ISBN 9781315673035 (ebook)
Subjects: | MESH: Mental Health Services—organization & administration | Practice Management | Mental Disorders—therapy
Classification: LCC R728 | NLM WM 30.1 | DDC 610.68—dc23
LC record available at https://lccn.loc.gov/2016017679

ISBN: 978-1-138-93588-4 (hbk)
ISBN: 978-1-138-93589-1 (pbk)
ISBN: 978-1-315-67303-5 (ebk)

Cover image: Photo by Olivia Ossege
Typeset in New Baskerville
by codeMantra

To our families, for all their patience and support of our writing and our private practice work.

Contents

Tables

Acknowledgments

We would first like to thank Anna Moore of Routledge Mental Health for her support and encouragement in writing this book, which began with a pleasant conversation on a beachfront sofa in Waikiki, Hawaii.

We are extremely grateful to our colleagues and dear friends who contributed chapters to this book, giving it a level of depth and expertise that we could not have achieved alone. Every one of them was professional and timely in all their interactions with us, making this project a joy to bring together.

We would also like to express our appreciation to the colleagues and mentors who inspired us in our private practice work: Robert Barcus, Ed Connor, Chris Dacey, Kathleen Mack, Rick Reckman, John Rudisill, and Janet Schultz.

A special thanks to the members, and fellow private practitioners, of the Cincinnati Academy of Professional Psychology, who so freely shared their wisdom and experience. Thank you to Olivia Ossege for her beautiful photograph of Alaskan waters used on the book cover.

Ongoing appreciation to our families:

Our children, Olivia, Evan, Jeremy, Ashlyn, and Caylee.

Our life partners and private practice business partners, Ted Ossege and Carrie Mason-Sears.

Last but not least, we would like to thank the thousands of clients whom all of the authors have worked with over the years, for sharing their life journeys with us, and for making private practice possible.

About the Editors

Jennifer M. Ossege, PsyD is the cofounder and managing partner of Viewpoint Psychological Services, PLLC, a mental health private practice in the Northern Kentucky/Greater Cincinnati area. In this capacity, Dr. Ossege oversees both administrative operations and clinical practice, while also maintaining an active client caseload. In addition, she serves as a core faculty member of the PsyD Program in Clinical Psychology at Union Institute & University, where she is the Associate Director of Clinical Training, coordinating clinical training, practicum, and internship opportunities for Doctoral Psychology students within the program. Dr. Ossege is also an Adjunct Faculty Member in the Psychology Department at Xavier University in Cincinnati, Ohio, and teaches in the Masters of Science in Organizational Leadership program at Union Institute & University. Dr. Ossege earned her Master's Degree in Clinical Psychology as well as her doctoral degree in Clinical Psychology from Xavier University. During her doctoral studies, her concentration was in child and adolescent studies and she also obtained a certificate in Organizational Concepts and Management. She is coauthor of the book *Hopes & Perspectives of Muslim American Women: A Paradox of Honor.*

Dr. Ossege is a licensed psychologist in the Commonwealth of Kentucky. After several years in private practice, she cofounded Viewpoint Psychological Services, PLLC in 2006, along with her partner, Ted Ossege. Viewpoint Psychological Services is a growing group private practice with three locations, employing several clinicians and support staff serving a wide range of clients in the Northern Kentucky/Greater Cincinnati area. Her practice website is www.viewpointpsych.com.

Richard W. Sears, PsyD, PhD, MBA, ABPP, is a board-certified clinical psychologist in Cincinnati, Ohio, where he runs a private psychology practice, provides consultation and organizational development services to businesses and agencies, and is the Director of the Center for Clinical Mindfulness & Meditation. He is also a member of the Clinical/Research Faculty at the University of Cincinnati Center for Integrative Health and Wellness, Volunteer Associate Professor of Psychiatry and Behavioral Neuroscience at the University of Cincinnati College of Medicine, Clinical Assistant Professor at Wright State University School of Professional Psychology, a member of the Affiliated Faculty in the PsyD and MSOL programs at Union Institute & University, and a Research/Psychologist Contractor with the Cincinnati VA Medical Center.

Dr. Sears is author or coauthor of *Consultation Skills for Mental Health Professionals; Mindfulness: Living Through Challenges and Enriching Your Life in This Moment*; *Building Competence in Mindfulness-Based Cognitive Therapy*; *Mindfulness in Clinical Practice; Mindfulness-Based Cognitive Therapy for PTSD, Hopes and Perspectives of Muslim American Women: A Paradox of Honor*, and *Cognitive Behavioral Therapy & Mindfulness*. He is also lead editor of the book *Perspectives on Spirituality and Religion in Psychotherapy*. He regularly presents on mindfulness and organizational development topics around the country to mental health professionals and the general public. His website is www.psych-insights.com.

About the Contributors

Kristy M. Fritz-Bosse, PsyD is a licensed clinical psychologist in private practice in Kentucky. She received her doctorate in Clinical Psychology from Xavier University in Cincinnati, OH. Dr. Fritz-Bosse received specialized training in a primary care, residency training program, as well as pre- and postdoctoral training in Pediatric Health Psychology at Children's Hospital of Michigan and Nationwide Children's Hospital respectively. Dr. Fritz-Bosse specializes in the treatment of children and adolescents with chronic health conditions. She has experience working with children with pulmonary and cardiac conditions, burn injuries, chronic pain conditions, feeding disorders, and other medical issues. She is also experienced in the treatment of other childhood issues such as anxiety, depression, and ADHD. Her clinical concentration is in working with children and adolescents; however she also has extensive experience working with adults. Dr. Fritz-Bosse is also an Adjunct Professor in the Psychology Department at Xavier University.

Andrea Schultz-Duncan, PsyD is a licensed clinical psychologist. She earned her Doctoral and Master's degrees in Clinical Psychology from the University of Indianapolis. She has experience in both inpatient and outpatient settings working with individuals across the lifespan providing assessment and intervention services. Dr. Schultz-Duncan's clinical interests include working with individuals and couples on a number of presenting concerns including depression, anxiety, health and pain psychology, communication, sexual health, and general wellness-based practices.

Dr. Schultz-Duncan also works as an Adjunct Faculty Member in the Psychology Department at the University of Cincinnati—Clermont College.

Laura Hensley, MA, LPCC has been practicing as a counselor since 2004. She obtained her undergraduate degree in Psychology from Hawaii Pacific University in 2003 and her Master's degree in Counseling from the University of Cincinnati in 2007. Laura has experience working with adults, adolescents, and children in both outpatient and residential settings. She has been in private practice since June of 2012. Laura Hensley specializes in the treatment of posttraumatic stress disorder, acute stress disorder, grief, depression, anxiety, personality disorders, and substance use disorders. She utilizes several approaches in treatment including Eye Movement Desensitization and Reprocessing (EMDR), Cognitive Behavioral Therapy (CBT), and Dialectical Behavior Therapy (DBT).

Joy McGhee, PsyD earned her Doctorate in Clinical Psychology in 1997 from Wright State University School of Professional Psychology. After completing her doctoral work, Dr. McGhee began working with a variety of individuals in both community and private mental health agencies, and opened her own private practice. Dr. McGhee's interest in vulnerable populations led her to spend 10 years working with children and adolescents as part of a school-based mental health program. Dr. McGhee has also served as Core Faculty within a PsyD. program, teaching and preparing new psychologists to serve individuals, families, and communities. Currently, Dr. McGhee lives in Cincinnati with her two teenaged sons and a feisty dog, and works with youth and adults involved in the criminal justice system. When she is not doing clinical work, Dr. McGhee serves as the coleader for the Cincinnati affiliate of the National CARES Mentoring Movement, serving the vulnerable youth of Cincinnati. She is also a regular participant in her long-standing (10 years) peer consultation group, which she attends monthly.

Ted Ossege, MSW, LCSW, ACSW received his undergraduate degree in Social Work from the University of Dayton in 1987 and his Master of Science in Social Work from the University of Louisville in 1988. He started working in private practice in 1991, and after working in several psychiatric private practices, he cofounded and has helped manage Viewpoint Psychological Services with his wife, Jennifer Ossege, PsyD., since 2006. He has helped oversee the growth of the practice from 2 to 14 clinicians in three locations, to become the largest private practice in the Northern Kentucky area. Ted Ossege has been a past item writer for the Association of Social Work Boards in Culpepper, VA, provides clinical supervision for other clinicians, has extensive experience in providing expert witness testimony for area courts, and provides training and workshops. Dr. Ossege is a former Adjunct Faculty Member at the University of Dayton, a Licensed Clinical Social Worker in Kentucky, and a member of the Academy of Certified Social Workers. He provides individual and family therapy to children, adolescents, and adults.

Emily Sander, PsyD, a clinical psychologist, earned her doctoral degree from Xavier University in Cincinnati, OH and works in integrated behavioral health at the Mayo Clinic in Red Wing, MN. Prior to joining the Mayo Clinic Health System, Dr. Sander spent her workdays at Viewpoint Psychological Services, a thriving group private practice serving the Greater Cincinnati area. She prides herself on being a passionate generalist clinician who enjoys providing individual, couples, and family therapy to individuals of all ages. In addition to her work in private practice, Dr. Sander honed her skills in a variety of treatment settings including hospitals, outpatient medical clinics, and the public school system. Dr. Sander incorporates learning and family systems theories with cognitive behavioral techniques to help clients learn how problems have developed in their lives and to learn new, healthier ways of living. Work-life balance is of personal interest to Dr. Sander, who spends much of her time attempting to balance the pressures of work, life, and the demands of a toddler, preschooler, husband, and two spirited miniature dachshunds.

Steve Sparks, PhD, ABPP, psychologist, completed his undergraduate education at the University of Notre Dame, graduating Magna Cum Laude. He received scholarships thereafter and earned both graduate degrees, Master's and Doctorate, at the University of Cincinnati. He is board certified in forensic psychology by the American Board of Professional Psychology. Dr. Sparks was formerly the Director of Forensic Services at Forensic and Mental Health Services, Inc., the state-sponsored forensic center in Butler County, OH. He is Adjunct Assistant Professor of Psychology at the University of Cincinnati (currently inactive) and the College of Mount St. Joseph where he teaches Forensic Psychology. His research has been published in the *Journal of Applied Social Psychology* and the *Ohio Psychologist*. He has provided psychological assessment services to numerous individuals, private attorneys, forensic psychology centers in Kentucky and Ohio, Ohio Attorney General's office, the United States Public Health Service, Bureau of Workers' Compensation, Social Security Administration, Catholic Archdiocese of Cincinnati, and the Bureau of Vocational Rehabilitation, among others. Dr. Sparks is a Past President of the Board of the Cincinnati Academy of Professional Psychology.

Heather Wilder, PsyD is the cofounder of Wilder Therapy and Wellness, LLC, a group private practice in Rhode Island. In this capacity, Dr. Wilder manages an active caseload in addition to overseeing administrative operations, credentialing, and clinical practice. Her clinical specialties include trauma, hypnosis, sex therapy, multicultural identity concerns, and work with the LGBTQ community. Dr. Wilder earned her Master's Degree in Psychology as well as her Doctoral Degree in Clinical Psychology from the Florida Institute of Technology. Prior to obtaining her Doctoral Degree, Dr. Wilder owned and operated multiple profitable small businesses for a combined total of 17 years. Dr. Wilder is currently a licensed psychologist in Rhode Island. Her website is www.wildertherapy.com.

Jami Wilder, PsyD is the cofounder and managing partner of Wilder Therapy and Wellness, LLC, a group private practice in Rhode Island. In this capacity, Dr. Wilder oversees administrative operations, marketing, and clinical practice, in addition to managing an active client caseload. Her clinical specialties include trauma recovery, grief, sexuality and gender concerns, and works with the LGBTQ community. She is also a board member and Early Career Psychologist chair for the Rhode Island Psychological Association. Dr. Wilder earned her Master's Degree in Clinical Psychology as well as her Doctoral Degree (PsyD.) in Clinical Psychology from Wright State University. Prior to earning her doctorate, she had an established career in corporate public relations and marketing. Dr. Wilder is currently a licensed psychologist in Rhode Island. Her website is www.wildertherapy.com.

Introduction

Jennifer M. Ossege and Richard W. Sears

If you are reading this book, you are likely interested in the potential independence, flexibility, and income afforded to those in private practice. You have witnessed time and time again the life-changing benefits mental health services can offer, and you know you have valuable skills to offer your community. You may be tired of being forced to meet productivity demands for an agency, or you may be frustrated by the arbitrary rules imposed on you by an employer, or you may have a novel idea to deliver much-needed services more creatively. Perhaps you are already in private practice, and want to get some fresh insights and perspectives on ways to improve or reinvigorate your practice. Whether you want to set up a full-time private practice, or simply see a few clients a week in addition to the other things you do, private practice offers wonderful benefits for us as clinicians as well as for the clients we serve.

Of course, embarking on any new venture can evoke fear of uncertainty, and freedom must always be balanced with responsibility. Those who are intolerant of risk, even when those risks are carefully considered and planned for, will always ridicule those with the courage to move forward.

We and our colleagues decided to write this book because we have all been in successful private practices for quite a while, and we enjoy sharing what we have learned, just as our mentors shared their knowledge and experience with us. Our editor at Routledge Mental Health was excited and very encouraging about this project. However, when we first submitted our book proposal, we were a bit surprised by the initial resistance we encountered from the reviewers. They expressed concern that private practice is declining, even though they admitted that they themselves were not actually in private practice.

Over and over, we've heard many people pronounce that private practice is on its deathbed. In fact, we first heard this decades ago in graduate school. Wild stories are told of how managed care companies or changing regulatory requirements have made it nearly impossible to be successful.

Yet, when we talk to our colleagues in private practice, and when we travel around the country giving workshops, people tell us their practices are thriving. We often hear that they have waiting lists, or even have to turn referrals away. This has been our experience as well. When you are good at what you do, people will demand your services. When asked why they thought so many people instilled fear into those considering opening their own practices, one workshop participant wryly remarked, "They scare you away from private practice so that you'll work long hours for low wages in an agency."

Working in a nonprofit agency serving others is a noble cause to be sure. There is also something to be said for job security, a steady paycheck, and good benefits. There are certainly challenges in private practice that must be taken seriously. It does take a certain entrepreneurial spirit, and a tolerance for risk and uncertainty. There are definitely legitimate concerns for those in private practice about such things as the ever-changing political landscape, the requirements of privacy laws, the hassle of dealing with third-party payors, and keeping up with the rapid advances of technology.

However, just as we teach our own clients dealing with fear and anxiety, if you want to move toward your goals, taking action and moving directly into the fear is the best way to deal with it. Compulsively avoiding fear only makes it worse, and leads to a restricted life. Of course, that action must be thoughtful and strategic, based on an understanding of the business principles involved in private practice, and weighed against your own skills, abilities, and desires. You don't need an MBA to be successful in private practice, but you do need to have or develop some level of business savvy. You may be a great clinician, but if your community doesn't know it, and you cannot manage your time and resources, you will have difficulty surviving. When we were in graduate school, alumni would sometimes visit our classes, and frequently say, "I wish I had more business training." The majority of mental health therapists spend at least a portion of their careers working in a private practice setting, yet most of us do not get specific training or preparation for establishing and maintaining a viable practice, much less ways to extend our career spans by reducing compassion fatigue or burnout. We intend this book to serve as a fundamental resource for mental health professionals, both new and developing, as well as for graduate students who are considering their career options. We also hope to inspire experienced private practitioners whose excitement and enthusiasm for clinical work have waned, and to inspire those who are pessimistic about the future of private practice.

In Part I of this book, we will explore the business side of private practice. In Chapter 1 entitled "Independent Practice and Consultation Services as a Solo Practitioner," Richard Sears explores a wide variety of considerations for setting up and maintaining a solo practice, including developing a business plan, finding a niche, and marketing. The chapter also presents ways to diversify income streams, such as professional speaking and consultation and organizational development work.

Since some clinicians may opt to develop or participate in group practices, it is important to consider the unique challenges and opportunities of this model of practice. Chapter 2 entitled "Establishing, Maintaining, and Growing a Group Private Practice" will highlight some of the considerations for establishing a successful group practice. Ted Ossege and Jennifer Ossege will share their expertise and the many lessons learned along the way in developing their multilocation group practice.

Chapter 3 entitled "Creating and Sustaining an Assessment/Forensic-based Practice" will address reasons why practitioners may seek to enter an assessment-based practice, and provides an overview of the types of assessments often completed in such a practice. Steve Sparks will discuss appropriate training, study, and supervision, as well as practical issues such as start-up considerations and costs. Potential pitfalls for an assessment-based practice will also be addressed, including issues of empathy, dual relationships, overconfidence, failure to consider alternative hypotheses, and sacrificing thoroughness for efficiency.

After a practice is established, whether solo, group, or assessment-based, success also depends on the proper management of nonclinical staff, and on the administrative tasks that are necessary to run a practice. This can be difficult terrain to navigate, and can be a challenge for the many clinicians who lack specific training in this arena. Chapter 4 entitled "Therapist as Manager: Supervising Nonclinical Staff and Tasks" will tackle strategies for recruiting, hiring, and managing nonclinical staff, including billing managers and support staff. Considerations of various models will be presented so that practice managers can thoroughly weigh the options that best meet their needs. Jennifer Ossege and Ted Ossege will also explore other professional relationships that are important to develop as one begins or grows a practice.

In today's private practice, the Internet and social media offer a window into the therapy room with a unique view. While the expanding technological landscape offers growing opportunities to reach and connect with clients, it also presents potential ethical and legal quagmires for private practice clinicians. Chapter 5 entitled "Navigating the Digital Landscape: A Practitioner's Guide to Moving Through the Rough Terrain of the Internet and Social Media" will present an overview of ethical and liability concerns and considerations for clinicians who are connecting with the public through the Internet and social media. Jami Wilder and Heather Wilder will review concerns for practitioners' websites, email communication, and social media sites, and will present strategies for effectively navigating issues clinicians are likely to encounter in a private practice setting.

Within the private practice world, clinicians must be adaptable, and be aware of the changing landscapes of service delivery. Forces such as managed care companies and the current political climate make it crucial for clinicians to maintain an awareness of the external environment in which they function, and to stay current on changes as they occur. Chapter 6 entitled "Integration of Clinical Healthcare Strategies: Preparing Clinicians for Shifting Roles" will discuss some of the newest challenges that are faced in the ever-changing world of private practice. As the need for health psychology services grows, there are opportunities for practitioners to expand their knowledge and skill-base into new methods of service delivery. Kristy M. Fritz-Bosse and Jennifer Ossege will discuss the importance of clinicians proactively positioning themselves as reputable, competent colleagues with an integrated knowledge base. This chapter provides guidance and practical tips for the clinician in private practice to enhance collaboration and improve patient care in the context of the changing landscape of healthcare service delivery.

Despite all the training we have received and all the tools we offer our clients, many of us don't do as well as we could in managing our own lives and finding a good balance for ourselves. In Part II, we will discuss clinician self-care.

Chapter 7 entitled "Isolation, Disconnection, and Burnout: The Importance of Staying Connected in Private Practice" explores the independent nature of private practice. For practitioners who choose this professional path, it can be difficult to avoid the experience of isolation, disconnection, and burnout. While many of us enjoy the benefits of being independent, there are inevitable moments when we face the challenges that come with such independence. Joy McGhee will address the benefits of participating in a peer consultation group and staying connected in order to build a sustainable career in private practice.

Finding an appropriate work-life balance is also an important part of self-care, and there are certain considerations specific to those in private practice. Emily Sander will explore this issue in depth in Chapter 8 entitled "Work-life Demands: Practical Tips for Finding the Balance," where readers will learn how to engage in structured goal setting, with the purpose of developing an action plan for the successful pursuit of work-life balance. The chapter will also address psychosocial and logistical issues that contribute to the perception of balance in the private practice world, such as boundary setting with clients and schedule planning.

Clinicians working in private practice can find themselves taking on multiple roles, quickly increasing the likelihood that they will become overwhelmed or burnt out. Chapter 9 entitled "Twenty-five Strategies for Engaging in Self-care" will provide reader-friendly descriptions of effective yet often neglected self-care skills to reduce burnout in clinicians entering the private practice domain. Laura Hensley and Andrea Schultz-Duncan will present practical strategies for self-care that the clinician can utilize to enhance individual well-being and contribute to the longevity of life in private practice.

It is important to note that this material will need to be adapted to the specific professional rules and regulations relevant to where you practice, and that even as this book goes to press, laws and technologies will be changing. Therefore, our intention is to arm you with general principles and strategies that you can adapt to the changing times and to your own needs. With proper preparation, you will be able to surf the occasional legislative and technological waves without being capsized, enabling you to then move toward your goals with smooth sailing.

If you have chosen the path of private practice, knowledge and planning will help you build and maintain a thriving practice that is resilient and sustainable over time. If you make the time to nourish your business, as well as yourself, it will be much easier for you to nurture your clients. The services we provide as mental health professionals are highly valued and desperately needed. We owe it to our communities, and have an ethical responsibility, to develop the skills to deliver our services as effectively and efficiently to as many people as we can.

PART I

PRACTICE MANAGEMENT

Nourishing Your Business

Chapter 1

Independent Practice and Consultation Services as a Solo Practitioner

Richard W. Sears

So, you're finally ready to strike out on your own, and hang your own shingle. Maybe you just received your license and have longed for this day, or maybe you are tired of working for someone else, twice as hard for half the pay you could be getting. Or maybe you just want to supplement your income with a small practice on the side, even for just a day or two a week.

Independent private practice can take two forms—completely alone, or alone with others. You could have your own private office space, or you could share an office with others. In either case, you are only paying for rent or specific services, and you are not subject to anyone else's rules or control.

Some prefer the structure and support of a group practice, which will be covered in the next chapter by Jennifer and Ted Ossege. When you are in a group practice, you can often rely on others to help deal with the business side of practice, but when you're going solo, it's all up to you.

Solo private practice is not for everyone. Even if other therapists rent space in the same building, it can be very lonely, since everyone is alone in their own offices all day. Those in solo practice like having their own space and independence, and find other ways to find professional support and connection (see Chapter 7 on peer consultation by Joy McGhee).

You will also need to have at least some degree of entrepreneurial spirit. In giving up the steady paycheck and benefits of a job, solo practice requires you to have a tolerance for ambiguity and risk. You will also have to be proactive to educate yourself about and take care of administrative and marketing tasks.

Some feel that managed health care organizations have taken away the freedom and profitability of practicing independently. However, there are a large number of clinicians who are effectively utilizing creative marketing strategies to maintain thriving practices. You can lament the negative effects of managed healthcare on private practice and give up trying to be independent, or you can take action and creatively establish a thriving practice.

You probably received great clinical training in your graduate program equipping you to deal with a wide range of diverse individuals and complicated presenting issues. Unfortunately, few programs emphasize the details of setting up your own private practice. Many clinicians actively shy away from matters of business, but when your livelihood and your family depend on your steady income, at least some degree of business savvy becomes essential to your survival. While you won't need an MBA to run your own business, you will need a plan.

DEVELOPING A BUSINESS PLAN

Too often, people dive into new business ventures head first and sort of make things up as they go along. While in some cases, this courage to seize opportunities is quite desirable and helpful, in other cases, it can lead to disaster.

Strategic planning is essential to any successful business venture. It involves clarifying your purpose, assessing your own strengths and weakness, analyzing the opportunities and threats in the external environment, choosing and implementing your business strategies, and monitoring and evaluating how things are going. Though plans should be reviewed and adapted over time, they serve as compass headings to keep you on track toward developing and maintaining a successful practice.

Before you decide what to do, you need to decide what you want.

Vision Statement

In the business world, a vision statement typically expresses the direction the organization wants to take over the next 5 years. It involves clarifying big-picture strategies. While your long-term vision may change and evolve with time, be sure to consciously pay attention to where you ultimately want to go. If you find yourself chasing after dozens of different opportunities as they pop up, you may end up losing your focus on where you really want to be in the future.

Before you can even begin to plan your business strategies, try to become as clear as possible about what you want your practice to ideally be. Just as we ask our clients, ask yourself what you would want 5 years from now, if you had that magic wand and did not have to figure out yet how to make it happen. Begin with a brainstorming session. Let your mind creatively think through what you would want if you had that proverbial magic wand. Editing your thoughts too quickly can stifle your creativity.

How many clients do you want every week? What kind of clients do you want to work with? What types of services do you want to provide? How much variety do you want in your workday or in your workweek? How often do you want to take vacations? How flexible do you want your schedule to be?

Your vision should include more than just your professional goals. Be sure to include all the things that you value, to build motivation to do the hard work that will come with building your private practice. One of my mentors, Stephen K. Hayes (2012), recommends keeping a document of what your perfect day would be like. It will change over time, but it can inspire you to keep focused on where you want to be. From the time you wake up in the morning, till the time you go to bed, what will your days be like? Do you want to spend more time with family? Greet your children when they get home from school? Where do you want to go on vacation? What hobbies do you want to pursue? How will you nurture your physical and emotional health? What do you want to do for fun? While private practice work can be very fulfilling, don't forget to enjoy your life along the way.

Mission Statement

Once you have a vision of where you want to be down the road, you will need to work backwards to develop a concrete, realistic, workable plan. A mission statement clarifies an organization's tactical plans, or short-term goals, typically for a 1-year period. It should concretely describe what you want to be involved with on a day-to-day basis for the coming year.

Keeping in mind your long-term vision, consider the practical short-term goals, such as making sure all your expenses are covered, and that you can earn a living. For example, your long-term vision may be to see 30 clients a week in your office, but as you are building your caseload, you might choose to adjunct teach at a local university, do evaluations at a local retirement community, and/or give regular public presentations to make connections in the community. If you don't plan your time well, and forget your mission, you may end up wasting a lot of time doing tasks that seem urgent but are not important (like checking emails too often) instead of engaging in tasks that are important but not urgent (like engaging in marketing activities) (Covey, 2004).

SWOT Analysis

Once you know what you want, it is important to do a SWOT analysis—Strengths, Weaknesses, Opportunities, and Threats (David, 2014; DuBrin, 2012; Whetten & Cameron, 2016). The first two involve an in-depth and honest look at your own personal strengths and weaknesses in the present, and the latter two involve investigating the opportunities and threats in the external environment that are likely to arise in the future.

Strengths

Begin by taking an inventory of your own personal strengths—the things you do well.

A good place to start is to take an inventory of your own character strengths using an instrument such as the VIA Survey of Character Strengths (www.viacharacter.org), which is a free resource and very user friendly.

Next, take inventory of your professional strengths. What do you do well? What specialized training or experience do you have? What populations are you passionate about? Over time, we can get so focused on our areas of growth, or on what we don't know, that we forget how much we really do know. You may be pleasantly surprised to realize how special you are when you begin to have people seeking you out for your unique talents and passions.

Weaknesses

It will also be important to honestly assess your areas of weakness. Knowing these areas will help you plan strategies to work around them, or at least to minimize the harm they might create for your business.

Again, begin with your personal areas of weakness. Do you have trouble getting going first thing in the morning? Are you easily bored by doing the same activity all day? Do you have trouble keeping up with details, such as administrative tasks? Are you comfortable with computers and technology? Do you have difficulty tooting your own horn (i.e., marketing yourself)? For example, I know that I simply don't have the patience to deal with insurance companies, and I don't want to take the time to keep up with the numerous and changing requirements of each company. Hence, my practice is entirely fee-for-service, eliminating the need for me to engage with insurance companies. While this may limit the number of clients who can work with me, knowing this about myself helps me focus on more fulfilling clinical work, such as personal growth counseling and organizational consultation, which are not covered by insurance anyway.

What are your professional weaknesses? Do you have deficits in your clinical training? How comfortable are you working with crises, such as suicidal and homicidal ideation? Do you have adequate training to assess for and work with the power and control issues characteristic of domestic violence situations? How competent are you to work with diverse populations? Have you been trained to work with all ages, or only a specific age range?

You may simply be able to avoid some of your weaknesses, as I do with avoiding insurance companies, or by making it clear that you only work with a certain age group. However, some areas you may simply have to work on, such as keeping up with the legal requirements of documentation or handling unexpected crises. While you may be able to make referrals when you feel that you are not competent to work with an unexpected issue that arises in therapy, incompetence to work with issues such as domestic violence could literally result in the death of your client and/or the loss of your license if not handled properly. Increasingly, clinicians are also getting reprimanded by state boards for working with cultural groups for which they have had inadequate training.

You can begin to address your weaknesses with regular consultations from colleagues, perhaps from local professional associations, or a peer supervision group (see Chapter 7 by Joy McGhee). Seeking professional consultation and continuing education workshops can help to ameliorate your clinical weaknesses. Sometimes technology, such as psychotherapy documentation software, can be helpful. Some services, such as accounting and collections, can be contracted out to specialty companies on an as-needed basis.

Opportunities

Once you have identified your strengths and weaknesses, it is important to assess the opportunities that exist in the external environment, in this case, the community where you will provide services. If you are conducting only traditional psychotherapy, this may encompass a fairly small geographic region. However, if you engage in activities like speaking or consultation, or provide services virtually through teletherapy, your environment may reach far beyond your local region.

If you have lived for a while in your local community, you may already be well aware of current gaps in services, and the opportunities that exist to fill them. Otherwise, networking will be important, both for assessing community needs and for fostering referral sources. Join your local professional association, attend meetings, and reach out to other providers. Let people know you are opening a private practice, and ask them directly what needs there are for services in your community.

To determine the needs that may exist at a regional, national, or international level, it is important to get involved in regional, national, and international professional associations. Professional publications and listservs often discuss these issues in depth, and can give you a sense of where needs and opportunities exist. It can also be helpful to approach experts in whatever area you are interested in, whether in person, by phone, or by email, and ask them directly about their experiences and what recommendations they would make to someone getting started in that area.

If there are already others doing what you would like to do, you should not necessarily give up on your plans. There is no shortage of suffering people in the world who need help, and there will always be opportunities for competent, passionate clinicians who do good clinical work.

Threats

Threats are potential environmental issues that could arise to create problems for your practice. Staying informed through local, regional, and national professional associations, relevant listservs, and business-savvy colleagues can help you stay abreast of changing conditions in the economy, laws, regulations, and with possible competition for your services. While you should not automatically despair when negative predictions are made, as they are often over-exaggerated, it is good to be prepared.

Once you know where you want to go, what you can do, and what the external environment is like, you are ready to plan the steps to make your vision a reality. You will need to develop both clinical strategies and business strategies.

DEVELOPING YOUR CLINICAL STRATEGIES

When I first began my private practice, I wanted to be all things to all people. When colleagues asked me what I specialized in, I basically said, "I do everything," and I wondered why I wasn't getting very many referrals. I specifically remember a turning point in my practice. I received a random phone call asking if I would do contract psychological assessment work for a company that did independent medical evaluations (IMEs). Even though I was busy with a teaching job, since my caseload was low, I began thinking through what it would take to get involved. While I had the necessary clinical training and experience, it dawned on me how different that kind of work was from the areas that were my real passions. I became keenly aware of the fact that even though doing IMEs might make me a few bucks in the short run, in the long run, it would hurt me by distracting me from my more important long-term goals.

While rural areas often need generalists, those in the city who say they do "everything" do not distinguish themselves from the hundreds of other psychotherapists in their communities. They also run the risk of spreading themselves too thin. It takes a lot of time and money to keep abreast of dozens of practice areas.

Having a specialty niche, or even several, provides a powerful marketing tool. Once I narrowed down my specialties to mindfulness, anxiety, and organizational consultation, I suddenly found myself with a steady stream of referrals.

On the other hand, you should also be careful about putting all your eggs into one basket. Some practice areas may be "feast or famine," so it can be helpful to diversify income streams. For those who dislike doing the same thing all day, having several areas of interest can provide stimulation and variety.

Managed care has eaten away at the profits of private practices throughout the United States. However, you do not have to be dependent upon insurance companies. While there are many thriving private practitioners who take insurance and practice in the "traditional" way, you should not automatically limit yourself to a practice based on the "medical model" of working only with those with serious mental health disorders. Our specialty is human behavior, and our skills are useful for a wide variety of applications, such as executive coaching, career counseling, enhancement of interpersonal skills, and development of parenting skills.

The areas below are meant to stimulate creative thinking, and are not meant to be exhaustive. Of course, as with any specialty, make sure you receive proper training and supervision before attempting a new practice area, and check your state board rules for what is allowed in your profession's scope of practice.

Psychotherapy Specialties

Due to the diverse range of human beings and the challenges that come up for them, there are many opportunities for specialization. Practitioners can choose to focus on specific age ranges, presenting issues, diversity variables, or a specific combination of factors. Sometimes clients and referral sources are seeking practitioners who are competent with certain treatment interventions, such as cognitive behavioral therapy, dialectical behavior therapy, or mindfulness. Some clinicians gain strong reputations for their abilities to work with couples and families.

Conducting psychotherapy in a group format can be more efficient and profitable for the clinician, and can be more affordable and effective for many clients than individual psychotherapy, yet this modality is often underutilized (Corey, 2012; Yalom & Leszcz, 2005). There are quite a variety of types of group therapy, from generally open personal development groups, to groups focusing on specific populations and presenting issues, to psychoeducational groups. Conducting groups can be more challenging than individual therapy in some ways. Aside from the training needed to effectively conduct groups, groups require more space, planning, and marketing. It can be difficult to gather enough clients who are available at the same time to begin a new group. However, it can also be a way to promote the rest of your private practice. I discovered that when I focused on running mindfulness groups in my community (Sears, Tirch, & Denton, 2011; Sears, 2015), it helped to establish me as a local expert, and people began seeking me out for other related services.

Take time to consider which populations you find most intriguing, and decide if you want to focus more specifically in your marketing efforts, and/or receive more training or supervision in a specific area.

Assessment

For those with proper training, conducting psychological assessments can be a specialty niche, or it can provide good supplemental income. For more about assessment in private practice, see Chapter 3, "Creating and Sustaining an Assessment/Forensic-based Practice," by Steve Sparks.

Organizational Consultation

For those who prefer not to see psychotherapy clients all throughout the week, organizational consultation can provide an interesting and lucrative alternative. As mental health professionals, we can leverage our understanding of such things as stress, emotional intelligence, systems theory, and communication to expand our influence far beyond the therapy office (Sears, Rudisill, & Mason-Sears, 2006).

When working with organizations, it is important to emphasize the bottom-line value of your work, such as how it will impact their ability to increase their revenue or improve their services. For example, working with a business executive improves the quality of life for that particular individual, but it also improves productivity through such things as improved communication and relationship skills. The popularity of Employee Assistance Programs (EAPs) attests to the fact that businesses are increasingly appreciating the value of the mental health of employees (Yenney & American Psychological Association Practice Directorate, 1994).

Organizational consultation can be divided into three levels: individual, small group, and large systems (Sears, Rudisill, & Mason-Sears, 2006). As with any new area of practice, be sure to seek out proper training and supervision in the area that interests you.

Individual Level Consulting

As consultants, we can work directly with individuals within the context of an organization. Executive coaching, in which the coach provides support and guidance to achieving personal and professional goals, is popular among those who wish to grow and develop (Coachville.com, 2003;

Kilburg, 2006; Peltier, 2010). Career counseling has also been increasingly needed, as young people seek help selecting a future path, or as older individuals seek out more fulfilling careers. Consultants can also assist employers in the employee selection process, to help them find people who fit the needs and the culture of their organizations.

Small Group Consulting

Organizational consultants can also work at the small group level. Instead of working with select individuals, a team or department is considered "the client." As mental health professionals, we can leverage our knowledge of group dynamics and effective communication to offer team building, conflict management, and workshops on a variety of topics, depending on the group's needs.

Large Systems Consulting

At the largest level, consultants can help entire organizations manage systems issues, such as planning and implementing changes, improving organizational communication (Conrad & Poole, 2012), and fostering a mentally healthy and productive workplace and culture.

Professional Speaking

While not everyone enjoys giving presentations, speaking can be a great way to share our knowledge and our passions with other professionals and with our communities. It is also a wonderful opportunity to position yourself as an expert and to promote yourself and your private practice.

Speaking for local mental health agencies and associations can be a good place to begin. Local organizations are often hungry for good speakers, and since many of them are nonprofit, they are very appreciative of professionals who give them their time. While you may sometimes receive a small stipend, the biggest benefit is the opportunity to gain new clients or foster new referral sources. Even one new ongoing client from pro bono speaking could lead to thousands of dollars in future income. Other professionals are also more likely to refer to you if they are familiar with your work and perceive you as an expert. Even if only a few people come to the event or training itself, you will often receive free advertising and publicity. If the sponsor gives you permission to do so, you can make a video or audio recording of the training, which you can post on your website to provide information to potential clients and to increase your credibility.

By performing specialized seminars for specialized groups, you develop a niche as being one of the only providers in the area qualified to handle such issues. Seminars are also a good place to gather qualitative data. By informally conversing with attendees, you can gather a sense of the needs of the community and what potential barriers there may be in seeking the services of a mental health professional.

You might also give public talks for your community. Organizations like the National Alliance for Mental Illness, Alzheimer's associations, and Rotary Clubs will benefit from your expertise, and likely lead to referrals.

If you like to travel, you could also join a professional speaking organization. Speaker's bureaus can match you with corporate speaking gigs, and professional continuing education providers can set up workshops for you across the country or even around the world.

DEVELOPING YOUR BUSINESS STRATEGIES

Once you decide what you want to do clinically, you will need to determine the best business strategies to be successful. This will include consideration of such things as incorporation, location, recordkeeping, marketing, and administrative support.

Should I Incorporate?

There are many factors to consider in regard to the legal structure of your private practice. Some general considerations are offered below, but be sure to consult with an attorney and/or an accountant about what works best for your particular situation in accordance with local laws and regulations.

If you have a full-time job somewhere, and are just seeing a few clients each week, you may not wish to bother with creating a corporation. You can report your earnings as business income on your tax return. If you wish to practice full-time as your primary source of income, incorporating can offer a number of advantages. For one thing, it separates your personal life from your business life. If set up properly, someone who files a lawsuit against your practice cannot go after your personal assets. Incorporating can also offer certain tax advantages, such as reducing your self-employment tax. Additionally, after you incorporate, you can receive an "EIN" (employer identification number, though you need not have employees other than yourself) from the federal government to use as your tax ID. You can use this number instead of giving out your personal social security number to the people with whom you contract.

While there are a variety of options for the legal structure of a corporation, many individuals in private practice choose to use an "LLC" (Limited Liability Company) or "PLLC" (Professional Limited Liability Company), which most states offer as an alternative to the more cumbersome requirements of a large corporation. Creating a nonprofit corporation may require more work than the typical solo practitioner is equipped to handle.

In solo private practice, you can simply use your own name, followed by "LLC," "Limited," or whatever terms are dictated by your state or local laws (mine is "Richard W. Sears PsyD LLC"). This makes it clear who you are, and can make it easier to set up things like business banking accounts. It can be awkward when people come to a place with a long name like, "The Institute for the Creative Application of Psychotherapy to Fostering Wellness in Modern Society," only to find you there alone. It may also appear odd to print business cards calling yourself president of a company that consists only of yourself.

In some instances, it may be useful to use a bigger-sounding business name, such as when you plan to develop a platform for a wider influence and presence, like leading retreats, holding classes, or teaching online courses to a global audience. In my case, I filed a "doing business as" (DBA) form with my Secretary of State for a small fee, registering "Center for Clinical Mindfulness & Meditation" as a name used by my LLC.

Setting Up Your Location

In addition to deciding what you want to do clinically, choosing where to open up your office is one of the most important early decisions you will need to make. While you can always move your office in the future if you outgrow your space, it is ideal to establish a long-term location. This makes it easier for referrals to find you, saves you the hassle of changing your address in dozens of databases, and allows you to get bulk discounts for business cards and letterhead.

You must first decide the general location you want to be in. It will be important to research the potential demand for services in the area, and what competition may already be present. Convenience for you (e.g., close to home) must be balanced with convenience for potential clients (e.g., accessible by major highways). If you offer specialized services, you may need to be centrally located, or you may need to be close to places like hospitals or clinics where your potential clients will be. If you intend to establish a cash-only practice, it can be helpful to research which communities have a large enough population and a relatively higher median income.

Next, consider how much space you will really need. Will you be working with individuals, couples, families, groups, or all of the above? If you do assessments, will you need lots of secure storage for your files, or will you store them off-site? If you are only doing individual therapy, you may not need much space. If you regularly do group therapy, you will need enough room to comfortably accommodate all the chairs. However, if you are only doing occasional groups, it may be better to share or rent a separate conference room.

Think through the other needs you will have for your office. Do you want to have a separate waiting room? Do you need space for a receptionist or administrative assistant? Do you need a secure records room? Is the space suitably safe, peaceful, and private? Do you want to be by a natural setting where you can sometimes take breaks, or see clients outside?

You will also need to decide if you want to rent or buy. If you want to have complete control over the property, and perhaps rent out space to other therapists, you might choose to invest in a small building or an office condominium. When buying, be sure to consult with a real estate agent, attorney, and/or accountant to consider all the ramifications, such as property taxes, condo fees, and depreciation. There may be tax advantages to setting up a separate LLC to purchase the property, to which your private practice LLC pays rent.

If you like the convenience of letting someone else manage the details and hassles of ownership and maintenance, or if you only need an office part time, you might choose to rent or lease a space. You could choose to rent space in an office with other providers, only paying rent and sharing common space, but still operating independently. There are even companies who specialize in renting out small offices with flexible terms. If you are only practicing part time, you could choose to share office space with other professionals. Of course, if you share an office, you must be mindful to keep your client files secure and your desk clear of confidential information when you leave (as you should always do anyway).

Once you establish your location, be sure to update your address with your state board, professional associations, Internet search engines, etc. Sending letters out to other providers lets them know about your new location, and will also serve to let them know you are taking referrals.

Billing and Recordkeeping

Your billing and recordkeeping needs will vary, based on your profession, legal and ethical considerations, insurance company demands, and personal preferences. Setting up a structured plan for billing and recordkeeping can streamline those processes and prevent problems from occurring down the road.

If you choose to accept insurance, you will need to stay updated on the requirements of each company. Many solo practitioners choose to outsource their billing services, and/or take advantage of billing software. For those who operate a cash-only practice, you could send clients monthly statements, or simply ask them for payment at each session. It is also becoming increasingly easy to set up systems allowing you to accept credit card payments.

Clinical recordkeeping is often simpler in private practice when compared to the requirements of larger agencies. Depending on your preference, you may choose to keep hand-written notes, use a dictation system, or employ software designed for those in private practice. As always, be sure to keep in mind the rules and regulations of your profession and your state board, along with applicable HIPAA and other privacy laws.

Your life will also be made much easier if you set up a system for business recordkeeping. Unless you are already an expert in business, it is well worth the expense to hire an accountant. Ask your accountant about the best means for keeping records for your business, such as an accounting software package, a simple electronic spreadsheet, or a hand-written ledger. Ignoring your accounting all year, then sorting through a giant box of receipts a week before April 15th, is not a place you want to find yourself in.

An accountant can also help you take care of payroll taxes and the payment of quarterly taxes, which will prevent hassles and penalties from the Internal Revenue Service. Also, because you are a business, be sure to take full advantage of all the expenses you can deduct off of your taxable income. Things like office supplies, continuing education training, and even lunch with professional colleagues may well be tax deductible. Set up a meeting with your accountant to make sure you aren't missing deductions—they could literally save you thousands of dollars.

Marketing

Once you're set up, you'll need to let people know you're there and what you do. There are nearly limitless possibilities for marketing a practice. In order to most effectively direct your efforts, a detailed marketing plan is essential (Ackley, 1999). It is important to educate yourself, develop short-term and long-term marketing plans in line with your strategic business plan, monitor the effectiveness of the plans, and alter or change the plans as necessary. Entire books have been written on marketing a private practice (e.g., Diehm, 1996; Grand, 2002; Steele, 2012; Stout & Grand, 2005), but the suggestions below will get you started.

Marketing for those in solo private practice differs from group practice (as discussed in Chapter 2 by Ossege and Ossege), as you are marketing yourself as an individual. Normally, humility is a valued trait, but if no one knows how good you are, no one will come. Though challenging for introverts, meeting other providers for coffee, lunch, continuing education workshops, or at local professional association meetings can go a long way to making those needed professional connections.

Word of mouth is the best form of marketing. When referral sources see the improvement in the clients they've sent you, they are likely to send you many more. However, word-of-mouth marketing takes time to get rolling. Typically, you will be most active in your marketing efforts when you first begin your practice, or when you expand your services, and you can usually be less active as momentum builds over time.

Develop Referral Sources

Recent research shows that direct-to-consumer marketing of psychotherapy can be effective, just as it is for pharmaceuticals (Gallo, Comer, Barlow, Clarke, & Antony, 2015). However, it is far more efficient to cultivate referral sources, from which a steady stream of clients can flow.

Mental health and other healthcare providers are always looking for good clinicians where they can send clients they cannot help. Take some time to craft a letter (or email, though letters are more personal and more likely to be read) describing such things as who you are, what services you provide, the types of populations you work with, what insurances you take (if any), and where you are located. Send it to colleagues, physicians, and every relevant referral source you can think of, letting them know you would appreciate their referrals. Though few may take you up on it, you can also offer to stop by their offices or meet them for coffee to get to know them and their needs better.

One of my first private practice mentors, Dr. Robert Barcus, instilled in me the importance of thanking referral sources when they do send clients your way. He said he was stunned at how often he would make a referral and never hear anything further, leaving him wondering if he was bothering the clinician, or if they really wanted the referral. With the client's permission, sending a thank you note keeps you in the referral source's mind, lets them know that their clients are being well-cared for, and that you are appreciative of them thinking about you.

Current and past clients can also be sources of referrals, because if you help them, they often desire to tell others about it. However, you must be cautious about the ethical issues involved in client referrals. To begin with, it is not appropriate for you to ask clients to help you with your business. Also, if you discover that two of your clients know each other or are related, it can raise sticky ethical issues.

Collaborating with local agencies and medical centers can also foster steady referral sources. You can offer stress-reduction groups, free talks, or as-needed consultation, which helps increase your visibility and allows you to establish more professional connections in the healthcare community.

Segmenting the Market

Segmenting and targeting specific populations and referral sources is important to maximize the potential efficacy of your marketing strategy. An undifferentiated approach, in which all community members are lumped together to receive the same marketing message, is likely to be inefficient at best. Segmentation of the community allows you to target the clients and referral sources who would be most interested in you. You can then approach one (a concentrated strategy) or several (a multisegment strategy) of these segments simultaneously or sequentially (Lamb, Hair, & McDaniel, 2012). As you know, all of our clients have both shared and unique needs. Typically, clients are divided into child, adult, and geriatric categories. However, within these are many subcategories, such as developmental disabilities, personality disorders, and neurocognitive disorders. The community may also be segmented by geography (e.g., city, suburban, rural), demographics (e.g., age, gender, income, ethnicity), psychographics (e.g., personality, motives, lifestyles), benefits (e.g., increased well-being, improved relationships), and usage-rate (e.g., those who frequently involve themselves in self-improvement activities) (Lamb, Hair, & McDaniel, 2012).

As discussed previously, having a specialty niche, or at least clearly defined populations with whom you work, goes a long way toward creating a successful marketing strategy. Think through your "elevator speech," the 30-second explanation you can give if someone on an elevator, or a colleague at a professional meeting, asks you, "You're in private practice? What kind of clients do you work with?" It's fine to start with, "I'm a generalist," but immediately follow that up with, "but I especially like working with ______ and ______."

You can leverage your specialty knowledge, skills, and experience by giving public and professional presentations on your topic, writing books, publishing articles in local magazines, putting out press releases, and by maintaining a blog or website with free information. Such strategies offer value to your community, and establish you as an expert in the field. They also tend to be more cost effective than paid advertising.

Make it Easy for Clients

It takes courage for clients to seek out mental health services. They may already be feeling overwhelmed by their problems, and may fear being stigmatized for seeking out services. Therefore, it is good to reduce as many potential barriers to seeking you out as possible.

Another thing I learned from my private practice mentor, Dr. Robert Barcus, is that if potential clients leave a message, it is important to call them back as soon as possible. If they get anxious waiting on a return call, they might change their mind about coming. They may also be going down a list of providers, and are more likely to make an appointment with the first person who calls them back.

A website with information about you and your practice, or a hard copy brochure that you can mail to clients, often helps them feel more at ease. You can even post a video introducing yourself and your treatment philosophy for those who are technically inclined. Clients can also fill out forms in advance to save them time, and you can send them clear directions to your office so they don't walk in the door feeling flustered after struggling to find your location.

Tracking the Effectiveness of Your Marketing

Research is an essential component in our professional training, and is important to apply to our marketing strategies. A simple line on the intake form that asks, "How did you hear about us?" can easily be used to track referral sources. If educational seminars or professional consultations for which you receive payment attract more clients than expensive newspaper or phone book ads, then obviously you should invest efforts and resources in the former strategies.

Bear in mind, however, that marketing is often like planting seeds. Someone who hears about your specialty, or attends one of your talks, might not decide to use your services until several years later when the need arises.

Ethical Issues in Marketing

Be sure to bear in mind the ethical considerations involved in marketing, in accordance with your profession's ethical and legal codes. For example, it is not ethical to advertise, "Your first therapy session is free." Clients are emotionally vulnerable. They may come in thinking they are only going to take the free session, but after telling their life stories and breaking down in tears, they may feel hooked into continuing even though they cannot really afford it. However, if the client is expecting to pay for the first session, but by the end you decide you do not have the expertise to help them, it is fine to say that you will make a referral and not charge them for the session.

For similar reasons, you should clarify your fees and whether or not you accept their insurance before the client comes in for the first appointment. Even though it can be awkward to talk about money with someone you have just met on the telephone, you do not want them to discover you do not take their insurance after they just trusted you with their deepest hurts and fears.

Likewise, you cannot advertise extreme statements like, "Guaranteed results or your money back!" Though it may be perfectly fine to reference research supporting the general effectiveness of the treatments you use, we can never guarantee results in psychotherapy.

The issue of referral fees is another area that can open up an ethical can of worms, and is best avoided. If you are giving money to other providers for referring clients to you, the providers making the referrals may be biased by their income potential, rather than thoughtfully considering what is best for the client.

MONITORING AND EVALUATING YOUR PLANS

When I do organizational consultation work, one of the first things I ask for is the company's strategic plan. In most cases, the executive has to dig through stacks of papers and binders, and dust it off before handing it to me.

The most brilliant plans are useless if they are never implemented. The best strategies may not continue to work in a changing environment. It is crucial to regularly monitor and evaluate how things are going in your practice. Of course, we already know this from our clinical work. We need to continually gather data and assess how the client is doing, and adjust our intervention strategies accordingly. We can use this same skill set to run our businesses effectively.

Private practice often affords you great flexibility with scheduling, which also demands accountability to yourself to attend to what is important. This requires you to manage your time effectively. It is crucial to regularly schedule time for yourself to work on your business and plans for the future, because it is all too easy to get caught up in all the seemingly urgent daily demands of your clinical work. Review your vision and mission statements. Take an honest look at your strengths and weaknesses. Update your understanding about the opportunities and threats in the environment. Polish your clinical and business strategies, and make sure they are still appropriate to the long-term vision for your business.

Of course, just because we are in solo private practice doesn't mean we have to go it alone. As will be discussed in Chapter 7 by Joy McGhee, it is important to seek out professional and personal support. Such consultation not only gives you emotional support, it provides you with an outsider's perspective on your business, and keeps you accountable and on-track with your goals.

It is also important to take advantage of other professional services, such as billing and collections, business and marketing consultation, and administrative help. A crucial concept in the business world is known as "opportunity cost," which refers to the opportunities you lose out on when you are engaged in another activity. For example, when you are first starting out, and have a small caseload, you might choose to do a lot of clerical and maintenance tasks yourself. However, once you get busy, you need to seriously consider getting help. You can hire someone for perhaps $20 per hour to do administrative work, allowing you to see another client during that hour for perhaps $120. Think of it this way—if you make your own copies and do your own filing, it may end up costing you $100 per hour. See Chapter 4 by Ossege and Ossege later in this volume for more considerations on working with nonclinical employees and contractors.

The idea of a solo private practice can at times seem daunting, especially when you hear the sometimes loud voices of the naysayers who fear stepping out of the security of their salaried jobs. But with planning and persistence, being your own boss can be incredibly rewarding. Creatively use the ideas discussed in this chapter as springboards for establishing your own unique niche services and you will become invaluable to your local community. While practitioners who are fearful of practicing independently stand on the sidelines, those who do careful planning, find the right support, and have the courage to dive in often have more income and more free time.

REFERENCES

Ackley, D. (1999). *Breaking free of managed care: A step-by-step guide to regaining control of your practice.* New York, NY: The Guilford Press.

Coachville.com. (2003). *The coaching starter kit: Everything you need to know to launch and expand your coaching practice.* New York, NY: W.W. Norton & Company.

Conrad, C. & Poole, S.C. (2012). *Strategic organizational communication in a global economy* (7th Ed.). Hoboken, NJ: John Wiley & Sons.

Corey, G. (2012). *Theory & practice of group counseling.* (8th Ed.). Belmont, CA: Brooks/Cole, Cengage Learning.

Covey, S.R. (2004). *The 7 habits of highly effective people.* London: Pocket Books.

David, F. (2014). *Strategic management,* (15th Ed.). Upper Saddle River, NJ: Prentice-Hall.

Diehm, P.J. (1996). *How to get more private practice referrals: A practical marketing guide for mental health professionals.* Garden Grove, CA: SCM Publishing.

DuBrin, A. (2012). *Essentials of management* (9th Ed.). Cincinnati, OH: South-Western College Publishing.

Gallo, K.P., Comer, J.S., Barlow, D.H., Clarke, R.N., & Antony, M.M. (2015). Direct-to-consumer marketing of psychological treatments: A randomized controlled trial. *Journal of Consulting and Clinical Psychology, 83*(5), 994–998. doi: 10.1037/a0039470.

Grand, L.C. (2002). *The therapist's advertising and marketing kit.* New York, NY: John Wiley & Sons.

Hayes, S.K. (2012). *The ninja defense: A modern master's approach to universal dangers.* Rutland, VT: Tuttle Publishing.

Kilburg, R.R. (2006). *Executive coaching: Developing managerial wisdom in a world of chaos.* Washington, D.C.: American Psychological Association.

Lamb, C., Hair, J., & McDaniel, C. (2012). *Essentials of marketing* (12th Dd.). Quebec: South-Western.

Peltier, B. (2010). *The psychology of executive coaching: Theory and application* (2nd Dd.). New York, NY: Routledge.

Sears, R. (2015). *Building competence in mindfulness-based cognitive therapy: Transcripts and insights for working with stress, anxiety, depression, and other problems.* New York, NY: Routledge.

Sears, R., Rudisill, J., & Mason-Sears, C. (2006). *Consultation skills for mental health professionals.* Hoboken, NJ: John Wiley & Sons.

Sears, R., Tirch, D., & Denton, R.B. (2011). *Mindfulness in clinical practice.* Sarasota, FL: Professional Resource Press.

Steele, D. (2012). *The million dollar private practice: Using your expertise to build a business that makes a difference.* Hoboken, NJ: John Wiley & Sons.

Stout, C.E., & Grand, L.C. (2005). *Getting started in private practice: The complete guide to building your mental health practice.* Hoboken, NJ: John Wiley & Sons.

Whetton, D.A. & Cameron, K.S. (2016). *Developing management skills* (9th Ed.). Boston, MA: Pearson.

Yalom, I. & Leszcz, M. (2005). *The theory and practice of group psychotherapy* (5th Ed.). New York, NY: Basic Books.

Yenney, S. & American Psychological Association Practice Directorate. (1994). *Business strategies for a caring profession: A practitioner's guidebook.* Washington, D.C.: American Psychological Association.

Chapter 2

Establishing, Maintaining, and Growing a Group Private Practice

Ted Ossege and Jennifer M. Ossege

Perhaps you currently have a solo practice and are considering growing your practice to include other providers, or maybe you are starting fresh and excited about the opportunities of establishing a group practice in your community. Either way, there are many things to consider when thinking about starting a group private practice.

As Richard Sears discussed in Chapter 1, many clinicians have extensive training in developing their clinical skills, without the know-how to build, develop, and maintain a thriving practice. Much of the discussion in Chapter 1 relating to clarifying your vision and your mission as well as analyzing your strengths and limitations apply here as well. Once you perform due diligence and carefully consider what you want, you will have a better idea on how to proceed. Some practitioners dream of a solo practice in which they practice completely independently. Others have a vision of developing a group practice, where a variety of clinicians can collaborate and work together as a unified entity.

For us, as we completed these steps many years ago and considered what we wanted to develop, we ultimately found we wanted to establish a group practice. Initially, we began very small, adding one or two providers as the opportunity for bringing on high-quality clinicians presented itself. After several years, our direction became more intentional, and our vision became clearer. Through this process we have learned many lessons and had many discoveries along the way, which we will share in this chapter in the hope that there will be a benefit to you as you set out to develop or grow your group practice.

Specifically, we will address the challenges and opportunities of creating a group practice, and provide practical tips and important areas for consideration while setting up and growing a successful practice with multiple clinicians. Questions to consider when setting up a group practice will be explored (e.g., forming a corporation, hiring employees versus hiring independent contractors, etc.) as well as other practical considerations. We will highlight the advantages and disadvantages of working within a group practice, as well as ways to grow a practice over time by steadily increasing referrals, adding (the right) practitioners to the group, and building a solid administrative network to achieve the goals of the group. Interprofessional issues (i.e., working with psychiatrists, medical providers, etc.) will also be addressed, since a focus on integrating patient care is becoming increasingly essential for good treatment outcomes (see Chapter 6 by Fritz-Bosse and Ossege for a detailed discussion of integrated care).

Assuming that you have gone through the steps of examination and planning set out in Chapter 1 and you have come to the conclusion that you want to establish a group practice, it is wise to consider how people will learn about your practice. Since your practice will consist of more than just yourself, you will have to find ways to develop a solid referral base to sustain a caseload for the therapists that you bring into your practice. Of course, some clinicians will bring clients with them, particularly if they have been in practice for a while. However, there are many times when clinicians seeking employment within a group setting may be just starting out and they have not developed a professional reputation quite yet. As the practice owner/administrator, it is up to you to develop a stream of referrals to help keep full caseloads for these therapists. This can be a big responsibility, but your employees will be depending on you to maintain their income, at the very least until they become more established.

SETTING THE STAGE BY BUILDING A REFERRAL BASE AND DEVELOPING RELATIONSHIPS

Growing and developing a successful private practice has its beginnings years before the first client walks through the door. It is difficult to imagine someone fresh out of school with no connections opening a private practice and expecting it to survive, much less thrive. The groundwork gets completed long before the first lease is signed, in the form of establishing and building relationships, attending meetings, networking, providing training, contacting medical providers, and establishing a reputation area-wide as a competent professional. When first starting out in private practice, we attended every school meeting about a client that we could (whether it was paid or not) to begin to establish our base of contacts and referrals. Some of the professional contacts we met at those meetings later became principals of other schools, heads of agencies, and colleagues in other practices—many of whom became dependable and steady referral sources.

We also gave pro bono training to state and community-based foster care agencies on topics we had expertise and experience in. We attended case conferences at different agencies about our patients, or hosted those meetings in our offices. In doing so, we developed a wide range of potential referral sources. One of the aspects of our practice in which we take a great deal of pride is the diversity of referral sources. We track our referrals by referral source, and find that no one source is dominant. There is a wide variety of referral sources, from previous or current clients, primary care doctors and pediatricians, school counselors, other practices, our website, etc.

It may seem counterproductive to "give away" your services through unpaid meetings, trainings, and the like. However, when you consider that an hour or two up-front often leads to either new clients or new referral sources, your short-term time investment becomes a steady stream of income, often lasting for years (or in some cases, as we have learned, decades). There are many ways to develop these referral bases, and they often begin with forming relationships.

Years before we even thought of opening a private practice, one of the contacts we made paid off in a way we never dreamed about. Several patients that we were seeing for therapy had been speaking very highly about how great their pediatrician was. They talked about how friendly and compassionate he was, and how he would go the extra mile for them. Thinking this provider would be a good person to get to know, we sent him a letter, telling him how we had been seeing several of his patients, how they had all spoken highly of him, and how we would like to introduce ourselves to him and his colleagues, and discuss how we could work together. Well, his patients turned out to be accurate in their description of him. He responded by calling as soon as he received the letter, and extended a lunch invitation to us to come and meet the other 12 providers (nurse practitioners and pediatricians) in his practice. He arranged the meeting so the majority of his providers would be able to attend, and we had lunch with them, providing a brief presentation of the practice and the services we provided. His providers were eager to meet us, and grateful they had a new referral source. We then also became providers that had a face to them, clinicians they could tell their patients they had met, which helps clients feel more comfortable about making the call to our office.

It needs to be emphasized we did not have our private practice at the time. This lunch meeting was 4 years before we went out on our own. The relationship was maintained over the next several years by providing frequent updates about patients. They have now become one of our largest referral sources, and since they now have 16 providers and 3 offices in 3 different counties, that relationship has provided a dependable stream of patients. Even with that, our referrals are not dependent on this practice. Due to the relationships with other entities similarly formed years before, we consistently receive diverse referrals from a wide range of sources.

Developing a Game Plan

What is your vision for your practice? Where do you ultimately want to see yourself in 10 or 20 years regarding your practice? Do you envision a large, bustling practice with several offices, numerous providers, and a large client base with many referral sources? Do you see yourself managing much of this thriving practice, or having others take care of the details while you continue to see clients most of your day? Or, do you see a small practice that is busy, but easier to manage with no intention of becoming a large enterprise?

If you want to grow, you need to be able to see yourself and your business 10 and 20 years into the future. There needs to be a vision, a sense of where this road is going, if you have any hope of eventually getting there. You will not be able to accomplish what you are not able to see, so take some time to think about your ultimate dream practice, and what it would look like. Create an outline of what you want things to look like every 5 years. This helps provide a framework for your vision.

Group practices, like many businesses, have phases of development. Initially, you work to establish the practice, referrals, business model, and procedures, which take up a great deal of nonclinical time. As time goes on, the practice starts to become profitable, and the referrals grow to the point where you cannot see every referred client. You face the decision to stop taking new clients and refer them elsewhere, develop a waiting list, or hire another therapist to share in the referrals. Once you start hiring other therapists, your practice begins to expand and develop.

But first, let's start with some of the initial developments of the practice. There are many decisions to make in the early phase of developing your group practice and therefore many aspects to consider.

Office Space

If you decide to lease office space in the formative years of your practice, and it has space for two offices, what will you do if you maximize this space in the next year, but have signed a 5-year lease? You may not have thought you would grow this fast, or even wanted to necessarily, but you would then be in a bind. Think about all the possibilities, good and bad, and have some sort of plan of what you will do if they occur. There will always be risk of course, but you want the risk to be somewhat manageable.

We opened our second office with only two full-time providers in a space that had offices for seven providers. We had already developed a solid stream of referrals, and we were confident that the location of the second office (positioned near a major hospital on a road lined with medical offices of different specialties) would be profitable, eventually. We also knew from our experience that it takes time for this to happen. When we opened the second location, things had been humming along nicely at the first office. We were able to pay ourselves regularly, were not concerned about our ability to make payroll, had enough money to pay our bills, and all was good. But our vision was not just for one office. We had a long-term plan of opening several offices, provided we were able to find the quality providers we sought. Our expansion plans have always hinged on hiring the right providers—not just good, competent providers, but exceptional providers. If we could find the right people, we could grow.

The second office then opened with only two providers, and with that opening came a large monthly lease, furniture expense, additional staff, and operational costs, and then it was back to where we were when we opened our first office, in a financial sense. We had to closely monitor our revenue to make sure we could make payroll each week, and expenses had to be kept tight. Our lease payment on the second location was almost twice that of the first, but two factors stood out that made this jump worthwhile. First, we were two doors down from the largest pediatric practice in our area, from whom we had developed a good referral stream, and this second office was located across the road from a large hospital and within a conglomerate of medical offices that lined this road. This location gave us tremendous visibility, accessibility for our patients, and some professional credibility as well. We were not a transient office that might not be there in the future, but a solid provider able to locate in an area with other legitimate medical practices.

We had room to grow in the second office, again contingent on finding those exceptional providers. Five years after opening that location, each of those extra offices are now filled with exceptional providers, we are bursting with referrals, and all providers currently have full caseloads. Our biggest problem has become managing the crush of referrals. Consistent with our vision, we are now in the beginning stages of opening a third office.

Consider what you want your practice to be, and plan for it. With a solo practice, growth is limited to what you can do with your time as an individual, but with a group practice, you can harness the talents of many individuals and work together to create something wonderful. This can be rewarding, but be aware of the risks involved, and make sure you are well-positioned before jumping into unknown territory. With each opportunity for growth, there is some discomfort. Those who can tolerate the discomfort, and can mediate the reasonable risk, can find reward in the growth of a group practice.

Naming Your Practice

Although it may seem simple, it makes sense to put some time into considering your practice name. Particularly as a group practice, you will want to have a name that can represent many different clinicians. Potential clients will begin to form an opinion about your practice from the start, so having a name that can represent your practice and clearly states what you offer is important. It is also important to think in terms of a lasting brand that you are creating that can withstand changes in location, clinicians, etc.

Many groups are named after the primary clinician (practice owner) and then add "and associates" to indicate that the practice includes other professionals. Part of every decision we have made in developing our group practice has been to take the perspective of other stakeholders, such as other professionals practicing in our group. By doing so, we considered the value of not highlighting our own names, but rather of creating a distinctive brand that allows multiple individuals to develop their practices and professional identities under this entity. We also considered a long-range plan of having a practice, and a brand, with the potential to continue even after our retirement. After all, what becomes of "Jones and Associates" after Jones retires? Another reason has more to do with overall philosophy and management style. In the past, we worked at a practice where there was a clear and obvious division between the owners and the rest of the practice. This division was represented in separate voicemail trees for owners and clinicians, a separate meeting room in the building only accessible by the owners, and exterior signage that only named the owners and none of the clinical staff. This left a negative impression, and became something we wanted to avoid in our own practice. If our group practice was named after us, then symbolically it would be about us, at least to some extent, and we wanted to avoid that implication, whether subtle or not. Our vision was to have a practice which was about everyone, with clinicians and office staff being just as important as the owners, and being treated that way. This name selection can be somewhat of a personal choice—there are thriving practices named after one individual. However, due to our past experience with the previous practice, we felt it important to select a name that was consistent with our vision for our practice.

Similarly, we also recommend avoiding names that include the city, or street, to allow flexibility if your practice is relocated to a different office space in the future. For instance, if the practice name is "Main Street Psychological," and you want to relocate to a different street, it requires a change in identity and branding.

Also, when brainstorming about the name of the practice, keep in mind staff who will be answering the phone. A long and clunky name that is time consuming to pronounce will not help with the growth and recognition of your practice. One practice we know has such a name, and in addition, the name is not descriptive of what they do. It is unclear from the name what kind of business it is. You want the name to tell what the practice is about, not make people guess what it is you do.

LEGAL/PRACTICE ISSUES TO CONSIDER

Before seeing that first client, or even hiring your first employee, you will need to consider a variety of factors to ensure you are establishing a professional, legal, and ethical practice. While setting up a group practice shares some similarities to a solo practice as discussed in Chapter 1 by Richard Sears, a group practice, by its nature, also has additional complexities to consider.

When we began making plans to open our own practice, we first met with an attorney to ensure we were going about it the right way and meeting all local and state guidelines and laws. We needed expertise on matters such as forming a PLLC (Professional Limited Liability Company), filing articles of incorporation, getting a tax identification number (TIN), and a myriad of other issues.

Will You Set Up Your Practice as a Partnership, Sole Proprietorship, or a Corporation?

There are many issues involved in setting up each of these entities, and requirements vary from state to state. One of the primary reasons business owners set up a corporation is to provide some protection from liability. There are different types of corporations (S corporation, C corporation, LLC, etc.), with different advantages and requirements depending on the structure. All of this information was well beyond the scope of our knowledge and comfort zone, so we relied on our attorney and accounting professionals to help us sort out these details. A CPA is also mandatory when setting up your own practice. There are quarterly taxes to be paid, payroll requirements if you have employees, accounting software to set up and be trained in, decisions to be made on how you will pay yourself, and regulations about the transfer of money between your business and personal accounts.

All of this can sound very overwhelming to a clinician who only wants to help people and support themselves doing it. The idea of dealing with all of the business details can be nauseating for many professionals. If that's the case, running your own practice may not be for you. However, one of the aspects we both enjoy about owning our own practice is having new challenges and variety in the tasks that we engage in. Posting payments on the practice software, meeting with our accountant about business expansion, or deciding on a new phone system for the office are activities that are very different from clinical practice, but can be refreshing and provide a nice change of pace from the normal practice of treating patients.

Will You Require Clinicians to Sign a Noncompete Agreement to Join Your Group Practice?

Before hiring clinicians into your group practice, you have to clarify your expectations. One discussion we had was deciding whether we wanted clinicians we hired to sign a noncompete agreement, limiting them from opening a practice or joining a practice within a certain number of miles of our location, if they at some point decided to leave the practice. We ultimately decided to *not* have a noncompete agreement, and admittedly this was against the advice of our attorney. Our philosophy was that if we treated the clinicians the best we could, paid them as well as we could, and avoided the owner pitfall of thinking we somehow were more privileged or deserved more than our employees, we would hopefully create an atmosphere where they would not be a big risk to leave, at least not to join another private practice nearby. Additionally, we believed it was not in the best interest of clients, who would likely follow these clinicians should they decide to leave, and we wanted to ensure ethical and respectable treatment of all involved. Ultimately, we realize that for providers to go out on their own is a huge financial risk for them, and many are not interested in running the business side of a practice. Sure, at first it seems enticing to keep 100 percent of your client fees. But once you start deducting the cost of office space, utilities, taxes, support staff, and other overhead, and add in the time that it would take for you to solicit referrals, manage the marketing, and other areas of a practice, most clinicians quickly appreciate the percentage that they receive from a group practice, which allows them to do the work they want without the hassles.

Will You Decide to Have Your Clinicians Be Employees, or Will They Be Considered Independent Contractors?

There are some pros and cons to both hiring clinicians as employees and hiring independent contractors. Let's consider the differences between them. If you are hiring clinicians as independent contractors, you need to issue a 1099, and the clinicians are responsible for paying their own taxes. There is no withholding, and the clinicians must make estimated quarterly federal income tax payments, social security payments, and state income tax payments if applicable. On the other hand, if you were to hire clinicians as employees, you would have them fill out a W-4 and you would withhold taxes and pay some employment-related taxes. Typically, the percentage paid to an independent contractor is higher, in our area averaging between 50 to 60 percent of revenue produced, compared to 40 to 50 percent for employees, to compensate for this higher tax burden. An employee paid at 60 percent however, will typically make significantly more than an independent contractor who makes 60 percent, because the employer will be paying some of the employee's tax, such as Social Security and Unemployment, which an independent contractor must pay out of their percentage. Most clinicians seeking a position at your practice will not be aware of this difference, so it is important to explain this so they realize that a contractor at 60 percent is not the same as an employee at 60 percent.

We know several independent contractors who were unprepared for, and also unaware of, the additional taxes, and thought they were making a higher wage than others in a comparable position, only to have a rude awakening when it was time to file their taxes. Be clear in what your agreement is, and be sure your employees understand how your practice operates.

One psychologist in our area switched his practice from having all clinicians as employees to having them all become independent contractors who essentially paid a flat fee to the practice. Each clinician kept all of their revenue, and shared expenses for things such as billing services, administrative help, etc. The rationale was that by having independent contractors, the owner was removed from the liability of having employees, and theoretically could not be held responsible for any actions by any of his independent contractors. Some clinicians may prefer to be independent contractors, if the collected percentage is high enough, but others will not want to deal with the added responsibilities of handling additional tax payments and would prefer to be employees. You will need to determine what is best for your practice before you interview clinicians.

Practice owners who wish to limit their liability may prefer to go the independent contractor route, while others who wish to emphasize providing a setting where taxes are paid by the practice may want to only hire employees. In our group practice, we have only employees. Our practice pays our employees at 60 percent of collections, while many practices in our area pay independent contractors 50 percent of collections, a very significant decrease in income for providers who choose to work elsewhere. It is not just a 10 percent drop, but even more when taxes and social security are factored. We choose to accept the additional risk in exchange for employees not having to worry about additional tax obligations. We feel the additional benefit to the clinician is desirable, and worth any risk to the practice to retain valued employees. This also allows us to maintain some control over the practice and to ensure quality control for our clients. While we do not micromanage the very talented individuals that we hire, we provide support and guidance when needed, and try to recognize their value to the practice. Since we all work under one practice name, our professional identities are connected, and we want to help each of the clinicians in our practice achieve their own professional goals as well. Along these lines, we require each clinician to maintain their own professional liability (malpractice) insurance. Additionally, all clinicians are included in our policy as employees, protecting our practice in the case where the provider and the practice would both be named in legal proceedings.

We recommend talking with a consultant, accountant, and/or an attorney to determine the best choices for your practice, and the implications for each choice. These are additional expenses of course, but well worth it to avoid massive penalties or legal fees later.

MARKETING YOUR PRACTICE

Now that you have spent time setting up your group practice, you have to consider how others will find out about your group. In Chapter 1, Richard Sears addressed marketing as it relates to a solo practice. Many of those strategies apply with groups as well, though largely the goal is not in promoting an individual, but the practice as a whole. Certainly, each provider can aid in this effort through providing presentations, networking, etc. But practice owners have the added responsibility of helping new clinicians with these efforts, often by introducing them to professional connections and finding opportunities for them to represent the group practice.

Since we have grown our practice gradually, we have spent very little on traditional marketing over the last 10 years. Our website is our largest marketing expense. We have also purchased pens with our logo on them, and we have had notepads made up with tear-off sheets that have our providers listed on them, website address, and a small map of our locations on the back. These are distributed to some physician offices, and are sometimes requested by referral sources.

The one factor we consider to be the most important to grow and maintain our practice, which many may not even consider as marketing, is prioritizing communication with physicians and referral sources. We utilize a very brief one-page form, which we send to the physician (with the client's consent). These forms can be sent for various reasons. Ideally, they are sent after the first session and provide a working diagnosis and a brief treatment plan. They provide confirmation a patient is attending, or notification in cases where the physician was unaware the client was seeking treatment. They are also sent when a client may benefit from medication, as in a diagnosis of ADHD or depression. Many psychotherapists are somewhat intimidated by contacting physicians, fearing they may be too busy or not interested in their input, but we find that most are very happy to collaborate and share information with mental health providers. While some of our clinicians are more comfortable sending written updates to primary care physicians and pediatricians, we have several clinicians that are just as inclined to pick up the phone and call. Again, the benefits of doing this cannot be overstated. If you have done your job in hiring well-qualified clinicians with good social skills, the impact of a physician having a discussion about a patient with a knowledgeable clinician goes a long way toward increased referrals. Some of the physicians we work with have even provided us their cell numbers so we can text them, and sometimes we communicate that way to arrange a phone call, or provide some follow-up. The whole team concept of medical providers and psychotherapists working together to help a patient is both satisfying to the providers and beneficial to the patient, and really speaks to best practice. For a more extensive discussion of ways to integrate services with physicians, see Chapter 6 by Fritz-Bosse and Ossege.

Many clients have long established relationships with their physicians or their children's pediatrician, and will trust their advice and recommendations implicitly. Imagine how an endorsement for a provider from a physician helps with the therapy process. Clients come in more prepared to listen and put their faith in you due to the positive information they have heard about you from their doctor.

As we talked about earlier, the groundwork for our referral sources was set years before we started our practice, with our prior experience in the field and relationships forged in court hearings, school meetings, workshops and training, phone calls, and professional networking. Had we attempted to start a private practice directly out of graduate school, the path would have been exponentially more difficult simply because we would not have had established relationships and credibility with our referral sources that soon. Much of our success was dependent on the legwork and hours put in during those earlier years, much of it pro bono, but it definitely was an investment into the name and reputation of our practice.

Without a doubt, the single biggest way our practice grows is through word of mouth. By "word of mouth," we do not simply mean satisfied patients telling their friends and neighbors about us, although that is a significant part of our referrals. We also mean satisfied patients and parents of those patients telling their pediatricians and primary care doctors about us. When a medical provider hears from several patients about the excellence of a particular provider, or practice in general, that practice can become their main referral source. It is remarkable to us that we have never met with or even spoken to many of the medical providers who refer to us. They are referring to us based on the endorsements of their patients.

It still gives us pause when we encounter a practice without a website. It is such an inexpensive yet effective tool for creating awareness about your practice and providing information to the public. It helps clients make the step from hearing about the practice to picking up the phone and scheduling. A website is mandatory if you want to create a thriving group practice. It gives credence and professionalism to your practice, in addition to being a tireless marketer. Our website has become increasingly important over the 10 years of our practice. We have seen the number of monthly "hits" or visits to the website grow from 80 to 90 a month to about 1000 without a significant increase in content, reflecting the increasing use of the Internet as a resource for people seeking mental health treatment. Just having a picture of a provider can be a huge advantage in having a client select your practice. If you see children in your practice, a parent can show their child what you look like, to help calm some anxiety about an upcoming visit; and for adults, having that image can help soften some of the trepidation that comes with an initial appointment. We have some brief research facts about the effectiveness of therapy on our website, some resources for different conditions, the ability to make a payment online with a secure site, and what to expect from an initial visit. We also have all of our office forms available for download by the clients, which saves us the time and cost of mailing out paperwork to new patients.

A provider need not be intimidated about creating a website. There are many website hosts that provide hundreds of essentially ready-made sites, where you simply add the content. The layout of the site, themes, colors, etc. are all completed, and can even be changed in seconds, giving the site a completely different look and feel. If you know how to attach a file, you can make a first-class website in minutes, with little prior computer knowledge. And you can even create a basic one if you do *not* know how to attach a file!

PRACTICE POLICY DEVELOPMENT

With a group practice comes many decisions about important facets of the practice, such as office space, which software to use, and more mundane issues such as missed appointment fees and cancellation policies. While we have attempted to keep our paperwork simple, certain policies of the practice need to be spelled out for your own protection, and for the knowledge of the client. We charge a fee if the client does not bring in the required copay, and we also charge a fee for an appointment that is missed or not cancelled with at least 24-hour notice. These are spelled out and signed by the client at the initial appointment. While it is not helpful to be militant about these policies, there must be some sort of structure to go by to maintain a profitable practice.

Take the copay for example. We know in advance what the copay will be for each patient, because we get their insurance information before we even schedule the appointment. Can you imagine going to your primary care doctor and not having the copay? It should not be any different for your own practice. We do see the patient if they do not have the copay, but we charge them a fee for not bringing it. We consider it a part of treatment to hold the client accountable, and we are not doing them any favors by letting them avoid normal obligations. Also, it requires more staff time to have to bill them for the fee and mail out a statement. The charge for a missed appointment or a late cancellation is $70, enough to make an impact and help the client keep an appointment if they are on the fence. Now, if a patient is sick, or the roads are bad due to ice or snow, or a situation is unavoidable, we typically waive the fee in those cases. It is generally left to the discretion of the individual therapist.

We do not currently use a collection service for past-due patient accounts. We have considered it and discussed it on several occasions, but currently have decided against using one. Part of our reluctance is a concern that using a collection service will increase the possibility of a client taking legal action against the practice as retaliation, and the additional concern of creating ill will by using such a service. Instead, we try to minimize the amount of any past due balances in several ways. Since we only use just a few Current Procedural Terminology (CPT) codes, and our practice software enables us to input the expected amount per our contract for each CPT code per each insurance company, we know what the client owes before they walk in the door. We check insurance benefits on each client in advance of the appointment, and most insurance websites allow staff to check the amount of any deductible that may or may not have been met. The staff then knows what to collect at each visit, rather than needing to bill the client for the balance, which is infinitely more difficult to collect. This practice minimizes client balances so that most bills are reserved for fees, such as for missed appointments or for not having a copay at the time of service. This latter issue occurs most commonly when a teen comes to an appointment by him- or herself, or a friend or relative brings a child to an appointment, and someone has forgotten to provide the copay.

However, we still try to minimize those issues by offering clients an opportunity to keep a credit card number on file that can be charged in those cases, helping them also avoid the fees. These credit card numbers are not actually physically kept on file; in fact, we cannot even see the credit card number. With written client permission, we are able to go into our credit card provider's website and charge a card that has been used previously by a client by only seeing the last four digits, thus staying within the newer credit card regulations and not compromising the data.

Occasionally, a client's balance becomes large, perhaps due to someone losing their insurance after the first session and not informing us, or confusion that may arise over what is listed on the insurance benefit page and what is actually paid, or a deductible had not been met when we were told that it had been. In such cases, we generally attempt to make contact with the clinician first to get some insight on the best way to proceed. The clinicians know the clients and their situations, and can best advise the billing department on how to proceed. They also do not get paid if the practice does not get paid, since they are paid on a percentage of collections. We want to make sure the clinician and the practice are both paid for their services, but we also want to proceed with compassion and understanding. Sometimes we work out a payment plan, sometimes the frequency of treatment may be reduced until the balance is paid, and there are certainly some cases where the client is referred elsewhere and not able to return to treatment at the practice until the balance is paid, if nothing can be worked out.

GROWING YOUR GROUP PRACTICE

So the practice you have created is now thriving. Clinicians are busy, the phone keeps ringing, and revenue is strong. Is it time to open an additional office? Part of this question goes back to your vision. How busy do you want to be? Opening an additional office is time consuming, and will definitely reduce the amount of income you can take from the practice while you are paying startup costs and additional rent. If things felt comfortable before and you did not have to worry about how much money was in the bank when payroll time rolled around, that will change if you open another office, at least temporarily. Ideally you will eventually be able to realize more revenue than before if all goes well, but there is clearly some risk involved in taking that next step. What leads up to that decision?

How quickly you grow your practice will depend on your goals, as well as the market that you are in. In our case, we began small and grew steadily. In fact, in our first office we had rented twice the space that we needed, with the intention to "grow into it," which we quickly did. As we grew our referral base, and our schedules began to overflow, we brought in new clinicians to help us keep up with the demand. When that new clinician gets a full schedule, and the client demand continues, then we add another clinician so that there is never a sense of competition for clients, and providers have schedules as full as they would like them to be.

The trick is getting the right person on board who will fit well into the practice and competently represent your brand. What is it that separates certain candidates from others? Of course they need to be qualified, come from good training programs, and have great references. But they also need to have a particular quality that we refer to as the "IT" factor, the intangible that puts them a step above other providers. It can be hard to quantify or describe, but it is what makes them exceptional. It is definitely a likeability, but also more. It is not just a warmth, an ability to make us feel comfortable (which in turn their clients will feel), but it is what makes us say, "Yes, patients will love coming to see this person. In fact, I would love coming to see this person." It is also an ability to engage a client right away, to put them at ease, and help them feel relaxed immediately from the very first session. It is not a particular personality—we have providers that are calm and quiet, others that are very high energy and perky, some that are straightforward and blunt, and others who can be very honest and direct but be so tactful the client really does not know they have been challenged. But all of them have exceptional qualities to their presentations that make them stand out, and all of them have the ability to quickly connect with a patient and make them feel comfortable. Of course, not every provider will connect with every patient, and we have patients that occasionally will want to switch providers because they did not click with their current one, but our goal is to minimize those requests by hiring providers that can connect with the greatest number of clients. After all, one of the most important predictors of success in mental health treatment is the relationship a client has with the provider.

Would you hire someone you would not feel comfortable coming to see yourself? Would you hire someone you would not feel proud to have a colleague, friend, or family member see? We felt it was very important that our providers pass that test, and we ask ourselves these questions throughout the entire interview process. Of course we are not perfect. There have been several occasions in the past when we eagerly needed another provider and compromised a bit on what we were looking for, and those clinicians ended up not working out. But we learned from those mistakes over the years, and became better at knowing what we were looking for. We will always try to make room for the right person, but we are patient in waiting for the right person to bring into the practice.

Once you have reached the capacity of your office, you have a decision to make. Do you stay steady and limit the size of your practice, do you move into a larger office space to have more therapy rooms to see more clients, or do you open another location? Go back and evaluate your original vision to see if it is still the same or whether there has been a shift. Make sure your actions are intentional and aligned with this vision.

For us, we struggled with the idea of moving to a larger space where all clinicians and staff could be in one location, or opening another location, making services more accessible for the community. Although there would have been a great deal of convenience (and likely reduced cost) to being in one location, we ultimately determined that we liked the small practice feel, and having various locations within the community fit better with our vision of what we wanted to develop.

An opportunity came along that we could not pass up. Somewhat before we were ready to add a second office, we were offered space in the same building as the previously mentioned large pediatric practice. At the time, we did not yet have the clinicians to staff an additional office, but we did not want to squander that opportunity. It did make for some leaner years financially at first, but we were able to gradually add clinicians, and it has worked out well, as we have had a constant flow of referrals from the medical community surrounding that location.

As your practice grows, it is wise not to add therapists more quickly than you can grow your referral base. You do not want therapists with empty appointment slots resenting the new therapist who is taking some of the referrals away. Although you may be tempted to offset your overhead of filling empty offices with more therapists, having many unsatisfied therapists will add more frustration than it is worth. It is best to ensure that your current professional staff have satisfying (but not overwhelming) caseloads before bringing someone new aboard (unless of course the new therapist is joining your practice bringing an established client base and will not be taking away from the practice referrals). Keeping an open line of communication and being aware of each therapist's current schedule (and their ideal schedule) will help you know when the time is right to consider adding new therapists to the practice. Developing a varied source of referrals will help build a referral base so that you can grow your practice at the pace that you want.

Ideally, your practice should be getting more referrals than it can handle before you open up an additional office. The exception would be if you are opening that second office in a location that will provide you with a steady stream of new referrals. Are the referral sources there and available in your proposed location? Hopefully you will already be receiving clients from those referral sources who will appreciate the closer location. Are there referral sources that you can call on, introduce yourself to, and take to lunch? As drug reps know, every medical office loves it when people provide tasty food! You will need the constant flow of referrals to support the additional location, but you will also need the clinicians to see them. Our biggest limitation to our ability to grow has always been finding enough qualified clinicians that meet our standards. The referrals have always seemed to be there, but we have only been able to grow as fast as we have been able to hire the right people. It would also be ideal to have a substantial amount of savings so you do not have to take out a loan for startup costs, as there are always unexpected expenses associated with growing your practice.

You should have some good data from your current office that you can use to calculate how much revenue you will need for an additional office to be solvent. You will know how much the average clinician will typically generate, can work up a proposed budget with the new rent amounts, and can use your current expenses to do some calculations. For example, we were able to figure from our current numbers that we will need a minimum of three full-time clinicians to make an additional location profitable. We can open with less than three, and will probably need to at first, but will also know that we will need to hire additional clinicians as soon as we are able.

ADVANTAGES AND DISADVANTAGES OF GROUP PRACTICE

There are many advantages to having a group practice. Some of the biggest include the opportunity for collaboration, decreased isolation, and continued growth as you learn from your fellow clinicians. We have monthly clinician meetings to share difficult cases, provide support and encouragement, and brief others on new information obtained at workshops or in conversations with other professionals. These meetings are important because even in a group practice, it is not uncommon to go part of the day without seeing a colleague, as you may be with clients at different times and not be free at the same time. We feel fortunate that our clinicians genuinely like and respect each other, which makes for such a nice work environment. (In fact, we fiercely protect this culture when it comes to hiring new employees.) Clinicians who like their coworkers enjoy coming to work more, are more likely to stay, and are less at risk for burnout. A solo practice can be quite isolating, without the opportunity for spur of the moment collaboration with a colleague, without built-in peer support, and without the energy that comes from having others working around you. Some individuals may prefer the isolated or silo approach of a solo practice, but it's important to consider the options in developing your practice.

Another advantage of a group practice is interoffice referrals. It is not uncommon to be seeing a child client, and the parent then wants a sibling to be seen as well, or the parent also wants to be seen. In a group practice it is easy to refer that client to a colleague within the practice, assuming that referral would be a good option for the patient in terms of expertise, and it is often more convenient for the parent, especially if they can coordinate appointment times.

Group practices tend to have more available resources. With expenses covered by more clinicians, we are able to offer a wider variety of psychological assessments, utilize state-of-the-art Electronic Medical Records (EMR) and other computer programs, and have office staff to answer the phone, return messages, and otherwise lessen some of the administrative burden of being in private practice. Solo practices may find it burdensome financially to provide some of these benefits without the volume to spread out the cost. In addition, particularly with larger group practices, having additional clinicians means more expertise in more areas. We have a clinician that specializes in eating disorders, one who treats sexual disorders, some specializing in trauma, several that treat couples, several ADHD experts, etc.

Certainly as an owner, a group practice means more revenue. If part of your vision is to eventually see fewer patients, and perform more practice management duties or even increase your available free time while still maintaining a decent income, then a group practice could be part of that plan. While expenses also increase with a group practice, ideally there will be a time when adding additional clinicians really will not significantly increase expenses, and then the additional revenue generated will be able to increase personal income.

As with all things, there is another side to the equation. As stated earlier, starting a group practice is not for everyone, and has disadvantages as well. By owning a group practice, you also take on more risk and aggravation. When something goes wrong, you are the one who is called. We have had to deal with issues encompassing plumbing problems, office floods, computer hard drive failures, day-long power outages, heat and air conditioning outages, and technology snags. Also, when there is an unexpected expense, it comes out of your pocket (whether directly or indirectly). As mentioned earlier, when taking a step toward growth there is more expense in startup costs for a new office, and there can be added risk in taking on additional lease commitments, furnishing the office, hiring new staff, etc. Having employees, it is essential that payroll is never compromised. You have to ensure that they are paid when they are told they will be paid. There have been several times (particularly early on or in growth phases of our practice) when there has not been enough money in the practice checking account to cover payroll or other expenses and we had to cover this from our own personal account, or take on debt that we did not anticipate. Often it is a matter of cash flow timing, but you have to plan for it—if it comes down to you getting paid or the employee getting paid, it's always the employee who needs to be paid. There is also the matter of ensuring payroll is entered in time to be processed, regardless of whether you are on vacation or not. We have worked on payroll from many locations while on vacation (including a cruise ship) in order to guarantee that our employees received paychecks on time. In a sense, as a group practice owner, you are never completely away from the business.

In conclusion, owning and managing a group practice can be very rewarding, as long as it matches up with your expectations of what is involved. While there may be less direct clinical work over time, there will be many other tasks that will require your attention. Being clear about your vision for your group practice will help you stay focused and attain your goals. We hope that sharing our group practice experience and the knowledge we have acquired over the years will help you carefully consider many aspects about the development, maintenance, and growth of a group practice. Whether you are considering joining a group practice as an employee or contractor, or establishing a practice of your own, it can helpful to take a behind the scenes look at what goes into a group practice.

SUGGESTED READING

Hunt, H. (2005). *Essentials of private practice: Streamlining costs, procedures and policies for less stress.* New York, NY: W.W. Norton & Company.

Paterson, R.J. (2011). *Private practice made simple: Everything you need to know to set up and manage a successful mental health practice.* Oakland, CA: New Harbinger Publications.

Steele, D. (2012). *The million dollar private practice: Using your expertise to build a business that makes a difference.* Hoboken, NJ: John Wiley & Sons.

Stout, C.E. & Grand, L.C. (2005). *Getting started in private practice: The complete guide to building your mental health practice.* Hoboken, NJ: John Wiley & Sons.

Walfish, S. & Barnett, J.E. (2009). *Financial success in mental health practice: Essential tools and strategies for practitioners.* Washington, D.C.: American Psychological Association.

Yenney, S. & American Psychological Association Practice Directorate. (1994). *Business strategies for a caring profession: A practitioner's guidebook.* Washington, D.C.: American Psychological Association.

Chapter 3

Creating and Sustaining an Assessment/Forensic-based Practice

Steve Sparks

WHY CONSIDER AN ASSESSMENT-BASED PRACTICE?

Since the coming of the managed care era of healthcare over the past several decades, reimbursement rates for psychotherapy and counseling have been declining (American Psychological Association [APA], 2015; Herz, 2009) and payment has become harder to collect. Although some assessment-based practices, e.g., some neuropsychological assessments, are reimbursed by medical insurance companies, this chapter will focus on developing and maintaining a fee-for-service-based assessment practice. Many of the assessments that are in demand from evaluators are via government agencies, be these county, state, or federal, and have no basis in insurance-based services. (The term "evaluator" will be used in this chapter to reflect that different disciplines engage in assessment services.) Medical insurance companies and managed care organizations are primarily in the business of providing treatment services, but may be willing to reimburse for an assessment if it provides a direction for treatment. However, there are many reasons for mental health assessment that are not based on treating illness. This may seem a foreign concept to psychotherapists accustomed to the medical model of treating clients with mental disorders for the purpose of healing. However, it is this same medical model that has, in the opinion of many practitioners, undercut the effectiveness of psychotherapy and counseling. This has occurred via a trend toward relatively permanent maintenance prescriptions of psychotropic medications, often in lieu of psychotherapy, and toward limiting the number of psychotherapy sessions that will be reimbursed. This is despite research that has shown psychotherapy to have the same or better efficacy than medication treatment for many psychological disorders such as depression (e.g., DeRubeis, Siegle, & Hollon, 2008), and without the side effects.

However, emerging from under the thumb of the medical industrial complex is just one advantage to developing an assessment-based practice. Another reason is to have the opportunity to provide services to a referral source whose mission you support. For example, the Bureau of Vocational Rehabilitation (a section of the Rehabilitation Services Commission of the Social Security Administration) provides services to disabled Americans to help them become employed and maintain this employment. Such services include job coaching, training, education, and helping clients identify reasonable accommodations to which they may be entitled at their jobs in order to maintain employment. For this referral source, a psychological evaluation is required in order to identify disabilities that are present, qualify consumers for services, and assess what areas of employment might be most viable for the individual given their strengths and weaknesses in the context of a disability. Many evaluators find this to be a laudable and beneficial service to citizens, and thus find contributing to such an organization rewarding.

Another benefit of an assessment-based practice relates to personality style. Some psychotherapists find that seeing client after client, back-to-back, does not mesh well with their personality. When I was in graduate school, I quickly learned that seeing clients in this manner was somewhat aversive and found myself hoping for "no-shows." Of course, all psychotherapists experience such a desire at times, but for those who have more pervasive feelings of this nature, an assessment-based practice may be a good alternative. In assessment, the practitioner is generally with the evaluee for a number of hours after which there may be an equal number or more hours spent gathering additional sources of data that will be used in conjunction with information gathered during the interview and testing session and generating a report. This work pattern of being with the client and then away from the client may be a better match for those practitioners with an introverted personality style.

Also, if one has been practicing in a hospital setting or working for some other employer, engaging in a private assessment-based practice (or any private practice for that matter) will afford a great freedom in scheduling and how one wishes to spend one's time. This is generally in stark contrast to the work/life-style of someone in another's employ. Obviously, in exchange, one will acquire a new set of stressors, most notably associated with lack of as predictable an income.

Finally, assessment-based practices can be quite lucrative, particularly if one manages one's business in an efficient and effective manner.

BEGIN TO BEGIN

The first step in initiating an assessment-based practice is deciding what type of assessment you wish to engage in. As you move forward, you may add different types of assessments, but each will require appropriate training and supervision. It is not feasible to hold oneself out as willing to do any type of assessment that may be available. Different types of assessments differ in the level of complexity and require different levels of expertise as will be discussed in more detail below.

First, a brief overview of types of assessments often completed by psychologists and other evaluators is in order. Keep in mind that a given educational level is often required per statute or organizational rule. The evaluator should become familiar with such statutes and rules prior to undertaking any assessment to avoid inconveniences such as loss of license. Many types of assessments require doctoral level credentials. The descriptions below are not exhaustive, and rather provide a very general overview of typical referral questions.

Social Security Administration disability evaluations: In these, the evaluator is required to provide an opinion as to whether an evaluee has a work-restrictive psychological disorder and the extent of impact of this on work-related capacities.

Social Security Administration vocational rehabilitation assessments: These have been described above and involve assessing disability and potential remediating services that will assist the client in acquiring and maintaining employment.

Bureau of Workers' Compensation evaluations: The evaluator is usually required to determine whether a mental disorder is present and whether this was a direct and proximate result of an injury incurred on the job. If such resultant psychological injury has occurred, the evaluator provides an opinion with regard to appropriate treatment and work restriction.

Veterans Administration Compensation and Pension evaluations: These involve a determination of whether a veteran has a mental disorder, e.g., posttraumatic stress disorder (PTSD) that is connected to their service in the military.

Pre-employment evaluations: These involve an assessment of whether the individual is able to perform the essential job functions of a given position. These are often requested for high-risk occupations such as police officers, probation officers, and firefighters.

Fitness-for-duty evaluations: In these, an employee has generally been placed on administrative leave, or such leave is being considered, typically due to an adverse incident that occurred on the job. The evaluator is generally required to assess the ability to remain at, or return to, work or what treatment may be required given the psychological issues present.

Clergy evaluations: Such assessments generally involve the determination of whether an individual is suited for religious life, has psychological impairments that may interfere with successfully integrating into this vocation, and whether an individual is a good fit with the charism of the religious community. (Charism is the distinct spirit, style, and mission of a religious community.)

Licensing Board examinations: Here, the evaluator assesses whether an individual has a psychological condition that interferes with his/her ability to ethically practice his/her profession and makes treatment recommendations.

Neuropsychological assessment: The neuropsychological evaluator generally assesses the presence and extent of deficits secondary to a brain insult or a congenital condition.

Forensic mental health assessment: Forensic evaluators usually assess the impact of psychological conditions on individuals involved in the criminal justice system or civil proceedings.

Child custody evaluations: Although a form of forensic assessment, this area warrants a separate category due to its level of risk and complexity, and the nature is self-explanatory.

Again, this list is far from exhaustive, and the descriptions above are gross generalizations devoid of the nuances of which practitioners in these areas need to be aware.

Different types of evaluations obviously have different levels of gravity and complexity. For example, Social Security disability evaluations are often completed in one session with the evaluee by employing a clinical interview of approximately 1-hour duration. Child custody evaluations, by contrast, generally require meeting with both parents, and potentially multiple children, and require considerable testing, gathering of collateral records, making collateral personal contacts, interacting with attorneys, and reviewing court-related documents. Similarly, there are varying levels of gravity associated with different types of assessments and different specific cases within those types. For example, an individual who comes for a disability evaluation may have already met with such evaluators four times before and been declined for benefits, and the report generated by the evaluator is simply one piece of data in a decision that is made by those in the home office. By contrast, a forensic evaluator assessing whether a man accused of murder was criminally responsible for his actions at the time of the alleged offense will be providing an opinion that may ultimately determine whether the individual is acquitted by reason of insanity or sentenced to the death penalty in some states.

Coming from a background in forensic psychology, when I was doing evaluations for one small agency, my reports tended to be long and detailed.

I spoke with the supervisor of this agency who told me candidly that, "You are giving us Cadillacs when what we really need are Oldsmobiles." I was doing more than the evaluation required. My choice ultimately was to focus on more involved evaluations that were consistent with my report style rather than changing this. These are the types of decisions that will have to be made as one develops an assessment-based practice.

PREPARATION

You knew this section was coming. Appropriate training, study, and supervision is essential in moving toward an assessment-based practice, and different levels of preparation will be required for different types of evaluations. For example, the American Psychological Association in their Ethical Principals of Psychologists and Code of Conduct (EPPCC) indicates:

> Psychologists provide services, teach, and conduct research with populations and in areas only within the boundaries of their competence, based on their education, training, supervised experience, consultation, study, or professional experience... psychologists have or obtain the training, experience, consultation, or supervision necessary to ensure the competence of their services, or they make appropriate referrals... (American Psychiatric Association, 2010).

Similarly, specialty guidelines also make clear the requirement of having appropriate experience and training prior to engaging in assessment work. For example, the Specialty Guidelines for Forensic Psychology indicate:

> When determining one's competence to provide services in a particular matter, forensic practitioners may consider a variety of factors including the relative complexity and specialized nature of the service, relevant training and experience, the preparation and study they are able to devote to the matter, and the opportunity for consultation with a professional of established competence in the subject matter in question...Competence can be acquired through various combinations of education, training, supervised experience, consultation, study, and professional experience. Forensic practitioners planning to provide services, teach, or conduct research involving populations, areas, techniques, or technologies that are new to them are encouraged to undertake relevant education, training, supervised experience, consultation, or study (American Psychological Association, 2013).

Standards for Education and Psychological Testing (American Educational Research Association, American Psychological Association, & National Council on Measurement in Education, 2014) makes similar recommendations. Most states have statutes requiring competency in areas of mental health assessment practice. As such, failure to acquire appropriate training may have dire consequences for the budding evaluator.

In addition to such professional and statutory recommendations and mandates, in fairness to the client, one should be more than a hobbyist. The evaluator produces an assessment report that will likely have significant ramifications for the evaluee, such as a receipt of the desired services, a receipt of financial benefits, imprisonment or release, or gaining or retaining custody of one's children. To say these outcomes are of vital importance to the evaluee would often be an understatement. There have been times when psychologists have called our practice interested in taking on some forensic assessment "on the side," to supplement their psychotherapy practice with the implicit suggestion that they feel ready to "jump right in" given their doctoral degree and treatment experience. I sense disappointment when we begin describing appropriate training that will be required. Consider for a moment your current area of expertise, be that working with victims of trauma, family therapy, or mindfulness for anxiety disorders. Surely you would not recommend someone attend a 1-hour continuing education course in this area, read a book chapter on the topic, and then provide such specialized treatment. So must it be for assessment-based services. Having taken a course on "Tests and Measures" in graduate school and having provided career counseling at the Student Counseling Center would not qualify one to then deliver professional assessment services 10 years postgraduation without additional training.

In this regard, appropriate preparation will differ based on the type of evaluation and level of complexity as described above. Such appropriate preparation might consist of completing graduate-level coursework, attending continuing education workshops of appropriate depth (e.g., not a 1-hour dinner conference), shadowing a provider who completes the types of assessments of interest, finding supervision, and completing appropriate self-study including a review of current research in the area. Another option, in addition to or in lieu of some of the options above, would be to engage in education by immersion. For example, if one were interested in becoming trained in forensic psychology, most states have a system of agencies, often through a community mental health system or state psychiatric hospitals, that provide forensic evaluations to the Court. Seeking part-time employment at such an agency may provide ready access to training, supervision, and continuing education in the area of interest that would likely be invaluable prior to striking out on one's own and completing such evaluations independently.

In summary, engaging in appropriate preparation prior to beginning or adding assessment to your repertoire will likely help avoid problems with licensing boards, allow for an appropriate level of expertise to be provided to the client, and engender a sense of confidence, comfort, and satisfaction in the clinician.

STARTUP CONSIDERATIONS

Whether you are currently engaged in a counseling or psychotherapy private practice, or are just starting out, or coming from a structure where you worked for an employer, the good news is that startup costs for an assessment practice are quite reasonable as compared with many new businesses, and are generally recouped relatively quickly through services delivered. You will obviously need office space, which can often be sublet from another provider. You will need psychological testing materials, which on the upper end of the expense scale may cost $1000 to $1500 per test (e.g., intelligence and memory tests), but will cost several hundred dollars in most cases. Expect to spend several thousand dollars to obtain appropriate testing supplies, including the tests and response forms. It has been surprising and disappointing to me to find the number of practices that use photocopied testing protocols to save money. Such standard practice is illegal and unethical, being a violation of copyright and most test user agreements. The dollars saved will not make up for the integrity lost. From the very beginning, evaluators should determine to manage their practices with the highest standards of honesty and integrity.

It is also recommended that there be some form of reception staff to greet your clients. Some practices avoid this expense by having a sign that greets clients who enter the practice stating that the evaluator will be right with them and to please have a seat. In addition to this being a rather cold reception for the evaluee, it may present other issues as well. At times evaluees will arrive with an entourage of friends and family who then will be waiting unattended in your waiting room. Such a lack of security and oversight lends itself to potential HIPAA (Health Insurance Portability and Accountability Act) violations, theft, and even vandalism. One colleague who used this empty waiting room method had the clock stolen off his wall. If hiring reception staff seems too much of an expense when beginning your practice, perhaps consider subletting or forming/joining a practice with colleagues so that such expenses may be shared. Obviously, you will need to obtain appropriate office items such as a computer for yourself, a computer (potentially a laptop) for clients to complete computer-based testing, a printer, file cabinets, etc.

As with any mental health practice, all materials must be kept secure under lock and key. It is beyond the scope of the present discussion to explore the nuances of remaining HIPAA-compliant, but suffice to say appropriate computer and document encryption is vital. Our practice has found the purchase of an Adobe Acrobat Pro (© Adobe, 2015) program, rather than merely a PDF reader, to have been exceedingly helpful with regard to encrypting digital documents received and creating encrypted documents that are not easily alterable by the receiver. There are many such computer programs and encryption methods.

ACQUIRING REFERRAL SOURCES

Note that the title above indicates *referral sources* not *clients*. In an assessment-based practice you will generally see the evaluee on one or maybe two occasions. As such, if you want a successful practice you will need to garner referral sources that can supply an ongoing flow of evaluees.

There are a number of methods for acquiring and maintaining referral sources for a mental health assessment-based practice. Since you have engaged in appropriate training and supervision prior to embarking on your solo practice journey, you will likely have made a number of important connections which will result in referrals to you. At the very least you will have likely gained insight into the structure of potential referral sources and how referrals are made.

At times, adding a referral source is quite direct. One merely places telephone calls to the various agencies, e.g., the Rehabilitation Services Commission, Bureau of Vocational Rehabilitation, or Bureau of Workers' Compensation, and requests materials to apply to become an assessment provider. You will have completed appropriate training and supervision by the time you engage in this step, and that will be important, because generally, such referral sources will require sample reports. With some government and corporate entities, the application process can be onerous and time-consuming. Some will require photographs of your office space showing that the facilities are appropriate and accessible to persons with disabilities, and others will require a site visit. (You may find yourself installing support bars in your office bathroom.) Some may require various forms of online training. Differences in requirements vary widely but are generally reasonable. Some sources will require that you possess specific psychological tests, while others will allow for your judgment in determining what tests are most appropriate for the evaluees.

As you work through what may seem like a morass of telephone calls, forms, forwarding documents, etc., it is important to remember that it is during this early application period that you are forming many of the professional relationships that will be maintained as your practice grows. Some of the people you speak to, although not clinicians, will be the ones making the decision as to whom they refer business to in the future. Oftentimes this will not be based on predictable or logical triage heuristics, but rather on who jumps to the scheduler's mind first, or evaluators with whom they have had positive contacts. In other cases, these are based strictly on location and scheduling availability. Nonetheless, it is important to treat everyone with kindness and respect, even when your patience is waning. You may find that there is a longer delay before seeing your first evaluee from the referral source than you expected which may be hard on your patience and your pocketbook, but in time the practice will come together.

Advertising

Oftentimes the best advertising for an assessment-based practice is word-of-mouth. If you are doing high-quality work, efficient yet thorough, using sound judgment and appropriate clinical tools, demand for your work will likely grow with little additional effort on your part. However, this may be accelerated by making contacts via local professional organizations and volunteering to provide presentations describing your assessment practice for little or no cost. Providing such presentations will have the added effect of thickening your resume and keeping you up-to-date on current research and changes in your specific area of assessment. You may be surprised at how ready and enthusiastic referral sources and local professional organizations may be to have you come and provide a talk regarding your area of expertise. Mental health assessment is a niche business, however, and such talks to large nonspecific groups, e.g., the Rotary Club, your local library, or at a church function may be less beneficial than more targeted, well-placed talks to relevant professional organizations and directly with potential referral sources.

Print advertising such as in local professional journals and your local telephone book can be quite expensive, but some practices have found success utilizing such sources. However, having an online presence has become a focus for many assessment-based practices, yielding excellent results at a very reasonable cost. In this regard, you will almost certainly want to develop a website. This can be done for little expense using a do-it-yourself template provided by many Internet server companies. However, investing a bit more capital by having a professionally developed website may be worthwhile. Once your website is completed, you will want to submit the web address to the large search engine companies such that when individuals are searching for mental health assessment-based services your site will have a better chance of being identified. Additionally, for often a generally reasonable monthly fee, such search engines will allow additional advertising on the top or sidebar of the search page which will feature your practice prominently. Paying for such advertising may also increase your priority status in searches even where your advertisement is not displayed. Also, some publications aimed at the general public (e.g., "pop" psychology magazines) may have their own search engine, and you may be able to advertise your practice via these publications, again for a modest monthly fee.

Such an online presence may attract appropriate and inappropriate business to your practice. (Recently our practice was contacted by an individual seeking a mental health assessment of their dog.) Nonetheless, web presence will attract appropriate business sources as well. Your website should also provide an online "brochure" where you may direct referral sources who are considering utilizing your services.

This is far from an exhaustive list of how to garner online traffic, but it is beyond the scope of the present discussion and beyond this author's knowledge to provide more technical information. Numerous resources for being successful in this regard may be found at the local library or through professional practice associations.

POTENTIAL PITFALLS FOR AN ASSESSMENT-BASED PRACTICE

Who is the Client?

Likely there have been many disapproving grimaces by those reading this chapter at the use of the term *evaluee* rather than *client*. However, this was quite intentional since the person sitting across from the evaluator (or his/her psychometrist) having their intellectual functioning assessed is usually not the client. This is a very important distinction between a psychotherapy practice and an assessment-based practice. In an assessment-based practice, the client is generally the referral source. The referral source will usually be paying for the assessment and will therefore "own" it. In many cases, the evaluee will never see the assessment and in some cases be prohibited from accessing it, e.g., most Fitness for Duty evaluations completed for public safety agencies.

A frequent mistake made by psychotherapists turned evaluators is being an advocate for the evaluee. As a psychotherapist, one is indeed an advocate for the client, helping them along to a path to health and wellness and sharing mutual feelings of satisfaction at successes and disappointment at setbacks. However, adopting such an attitude is dangerous ground for the assessment specialist, who may at times provide opinions that are contrary to the well-being of the client, at least from the evaluee's perspective. For example, the evaluee may state that he experiences anxiety caused by a work-related industrial injury and deserves benefits to be paid him since this interferes with his ability to function presently. However, you may determine that his experience of anxiety predates the work-related injury and his current symptomatology is not a direct and proximate result of that injury. I have reviewed many a report in which the provider appears willing to bend the facts a bit in order to suit the needs of the evaluee because they view themselves as a helping professional and want to satisfy the evaluee before them. This is indeed a grave error and the beginning of a slippery slope in which the evaluator's integrity is again compromised and his or her opinion, in not only that case but in future cases, becomes suspect.

In forming an opinion, the evaluator must consider various hypotheses, e.g., the evaluee's perspective and the employer's perspective, but must come to a conclusion based on the preponderance of the available evidence and provide that opinion even if it is contrary to what the evaluator thought or even hoped would happen. In stating this opinion, one may also recognize potential alternative hypotheses. Packer (2009) has suggested that every report have a section explicating the most likely alternative hypothesis to that provided and then explain why the chosen hypothesis appears more likely. This seems like a good practice and is encouraged.

Clinicians who have developed a tendency to bend their opinions in a manner to suit their own needs, the needs of the evaluee, or their referral source have been referred to as *objectively impaired clinicians* (Zusman & Simon, 1983). Another form of objective impairment is when a given referral source, such as a lawyer or employer, advocates a certain outcome to the evaluation and the evaluator then considers this hypothesis above others and favors it due to the preexisting relationship with the referral source. Some referring parties may not provide future referrals if the evaluator provides opinions contrary to those advocated or expected. If you intend to develop an assessment-based practice it is essential that this eventuality be accepted. There are times you will lose business and thus income due to maintaining an ethical practice. This will occur. The evaluator must expect it and mentally prepare for it. Know that you are the more ethical clinician and better person for eschewing higher income (at least in the short run) in order to maintain your objectivity.

For those engaged in assessment practice, the names of those who are objectively impaired in their locality in their specialty are well known. The ethical evaluator may take pride in knowing that although their income may be a bit lower, they are not on that list. I will restate for emphasis, if you do not believe that you have the willpower to avoid having your opinion swayed by having heartstrings pulled by an evaluee or purse strings pulled by a referral source, it is important that you not enter the field of mental health assessment so as to allow for the integrity of the field as a whole.

Empathy

Wrong. This section does not explain the importance of empathy in assessment. Rather, contrary to a psychotherapeutic relationship, during the assessment of an evaluee, being overly empathic can be deceptive and counterproductive. It suggests to the evaluee that the evaluator is an advocate there to help them and this is not the case. The evaluator's function, rather, is to provide an objective assessment that may or may not be helpful to the evaluee. On many occasions in my career, after having painstakingly explained the nature of the evaluator-evaluee relationship and the purpose of the evaluation, at some point during the interview the evaluee will make a statement such as, "I know I need to tell you this because I know you're just here to help me." The evaluee has defaulted to this position because traditionally this is the nature of the mental health professional relationship with the person sitting across from them. Such misconceptions must be immediately corrected and again made clear that the results of the assessment will be objective, that these may or may not be beneficial to them, and that the evaluator is not an advocate for their position. This is not to say that one cannot make an occasional statement that is supportive of one made by the evaluee, or build rapport by engaging in some small talk conversation. However, anything more than that implies a relationship that does not exist and this is unfair and misleading to the evaluee.

Dual Relationships

Some psychotherapists who have added assessment to their practice believe a logical step is to provide assessment services to their current psychotherapy clients. However, this is to be avoided. Again, the nature of the psychotherapy relationship is advocacy, while the nature of the assessment relationship is objectivity. It is extremely difficult to adequately maintain both roles with one client. The professional literature suggests the same. For example, Heilbrun, Grisso, and Goldstein (2009) suggest that taking on both roles may negatively influence objectivity, interfere with adequate performance of both roles, and that the assessment role may negatively affect the treatment relationship. Rather, if your psychotherapy client is in need of assessment services, it is better to refer him/her to another professional. In one case, a professional decided that her psychotherapy client was clearly the most appropriate custodial parent to be chosen in a divorce proceeding based on what she knew of her client and what her client had told her about her client's former husband. She therefore provided a very one-sided, nonobjective custody evaluation to the Court. These types of dual relationships are to be avoided in the interests of objectivity, integrity, and fair dealing with the Court and all participants involved in a proceeding.

Overconfidence

Over time, some evaluators become overconfident in their intuitive powers, and begin to rely more on subjective appraisal than other forms of data. In other words, they start to "shoot from the hip," providing opinions that rely almost solely on clinical judgment and observation. They may jump to conclusions too quickly. Research has shown that clinical judgment may be faulty and that objective data is often superior to the practitioner's opinion based on "years of experience" (Grove & Lloyd, 2006). Avoid the overconfidence pitfall by maintaining humility, and adopting a thorough multimethod hypothesis-testing approach to assessment (both discussed below).

Failure to Consider Alternative Hypotheses

Generally during an assessment, but at times prior to this, the evaluator will develop hypotheses as to the answer to a given referral question. The evaluator may then seek information that will confirm their hypotheses, which is acceptable, but may find themselves dismissing disconfirming information, which is not. The evaluator should rather keep an open mind and remain flexible and willing to discard a working hypothesis when the data no longer supports this. The evaluator should at least consider other hypotheses simultaneously. Oftentimes Occam's Razor is an appropriate hypothesis-pairing tool, that is, acceptance of the most obvious and simple answer consistent with the data. However, at other times, cases will be more complex and require further investigation by the evaluator. The evaluator must be willing to take these extra steps when necessary despite a desire to maintain an already formulated opinion that could be dictated into a report prior to the arrival of the evaluator's next appointment.

Sacrificing Thoroughness for Efficiency

Although this is generally self-explanatory, I will note that there is often a tendency to want to complete a report in a short period of time, particularly if one is being paid a flat rate rather than an hourly rate. However, thoroughness is essential and must be maintained despite the effect this may have on one's bottom line or schedule. In addition to being the right thing to do ethically, it may also save the embarrassment that occurs when additional opinion-changing data is raised by another party at a later date. If the evaluator had only requested those records, called that collateral source, given one more test, etc., the opinion would not have been shown to be suspect.

A FEW WORDS ON MALINGERING

Malingering is the intentional production of false or grossly exaggerated symptoms motivated by external incentives (American Psychiatric Association, 2013). *Feigning* is a term often used to suggest malingering but where the evaluator does not have sufficient information to attribute the fabrication of symptoms to specific external incentives, i.e., secondary gain.

Exaggeration, embellishment, and *overreporting,* rather, suggest that the evaluee has some legitimate symptoms but is describing these in a less than accurate manner, although perhaps not rising to the level of "gross exaggeration." This tendency is of great concern to the evaluator as there is frequently the potential for secondary gain to the evaluee, including monetary awards, benefits, potential to be prescribed medication including controlled substances, and the mitigation of responsibility for illegal behaviors.

However, it is important to recognize that all mental health specialists, whether they be psychotherapists, counselors, or evaluators, should concern themselves with this issue. It is much to the chagrin of many assessment-based evaluators to suspect malingering and receive compelling support for this hypothesis from the results of psychological testing and other sources, only to request and receive collateral records from a counselor or other mental health professional who has clearly not taken this potentiality into consideration. To some degree this is understandable, as the counselor or psychotherapist rightly may see themselves as an advocate and so is likely to be more accepting of the self-report of their client. However, to provide counseling or psychotherapy services to heal an illness that does not exist is at best a waste of time and resources and at worst an ethical violation if this should have been recognized. As described above, there are many reasons that individuals may come to seek psychotherapy, counseling, psychiatric treatment, or even psychiatric hospitalization that are for purposes other than addressing legitimate symptoms.

Research has shown that feigning or malingering behavior occurs at different rates in different areas of mental health practice. Some research (in Rogers, 2008) found malingering rates ranging from 7 percent to 17 percent in psychological evaluations, and other estimates have been higher. Malingering should be considered in all areas of mental health practice, but is of particular importance for the evaluating psychologist. Many psychotherapists and counselors, and some evaluators, particularly those new to the area, feel uncomfortable indicating in a report that an evaluee has not been honest or have presented alleged symptoms in a deceptive manner. However, of utmost importance is that the evaluator provide the most accurate and objective report that they are able to give and that they describe their findings in an unbiased manner. This imperative should override feelings of discomfort.

There are a number of ways that the evaluator may address this difficult issue. Well-validated objective testing is available in this regard. In fact, some have argued that if one does not include objective testing of response style and symptom exaggeration the evaluator must have strong justification for having omitted this. Additionally, there are subjective signs of exaggeration, such as atypical descriptions of symptoms, frequent, "I don't know," responses, extreme symptom reports, inconsistencies in statements to different providers, and inconsistency between reported symptoms and observed behaviors. This is not an exhaustive list, and the prospective evaluator is recommended to become familiarized with the substantial literature in this area (e.g., McCarthy-Jones & Resnick, 2014; Rogers, 2008).

MULTIMETHOD APPROACH TO ASSESSMENT

As discussed, practitioners often rely on their clinical judgment in coming to conclusions in mental health assessments. Indeed, good clinical judgment and observation are vital, but must be only part of the assessment process. Experts in the field of assessment have generally advised that using a multimethod approach to assessment yields more valid results (e.g., Heilbrun, Grisso, & Goldstein, 2009). The following sources of information should generally be included in the assessment procedure.

Self-Report

An evaluee's self-report of his symptoms and functioning is an important source of data. The evaluator will want to take a detailed history in order to assess how past experiences may influence current mental status and functioning and also take a detailed account of self-reported symptoms going through each major symptom group in the *Diagnostic and Statistical Manual, 5th Edition* (American Psychiatric Association, 2013).

Observation

Assessment reports should generally have a mental status section in which a description of how the evaluee presented is detailed. Most mental status evaluations include a description of appearance, orientation, speech (rate, rhythm, and volume), eye contact, any unusual motor activity, mood (described by evaluee), affect (observed), reported suicidality or homicidality, thought process (e.g., tangential, circumstantial), thought content (e.g., delusions), other psychoses (e.g., hallucinations or overt lack of contact with reality), attention/concentration, memory, cooperation level, insight into symptoms, social judgment, abstraction (e.g., hypothetical reasoning), intellectual functioning (e.g., "grossly normal" or "potentially below the norm" if not tested), and medications taken the day of the evaluation.

Psychological Testing

Objective data is an important part of the assessment process. What tests are chosen will usually depend on the referral question, the evaluee's history, and observations made during the clinical interview. Research has suggested that the results of psychological testing may be more valid in assessing an evaluee's mental state than is the clinician's clinical judgment (Grove & Lloyd, 2006). When choosing psychological testing, the evaluator should bear in mind the referral question at hand and choose a psychological test that appropriately addresses the question. A "one-size-fits-all" method of psychological testing is usually not the most judicious or parsimonious technique (although such a method has been recommended in some cases for neuropsychological analysis).

It is important that the evaluator bear in mind that the tests chosen have appropriate reliability and validity rates and are generally accepted in the field. Indeed, such factors are generally required for evaluation results to be admissible in court (Daubert v. Merrell Dow Pharmaceuticals, Inc., 1993). Even if you do not intend to engage in forensic mental health assessment, most assessments have some intersection with the legal system, and the evaluator would be well advised to have used methods that meet these acceptable legal standards.

Beyond any legal ramifications, it is simply good practice to use tests that are reliable, valid, and accepted. In many niche areas of an assessment practice, there is research indicating which tests are used most frequently by evaluators addressing the referral question. As an example, Archer et al. (2006) have provided data from a survey of board certified forensic psychologists for use in the most common forensic evaluations. Similar studies have been done with regard to child custody evaluations (Bow, Gould, Flens, & Greenhut, 2010), neuropsychological evaluations (Rabin, Barr, & Burton, 2005), and other areas of assessment. Additionally, *Buros Mental Measurements Yearbook* (Buros Center, 2014) is a good source for psychological testing reviews, and inclusion in this publication suggests some level of acceptance in the field. Evaluators should be familiar with the Standards for Educational and Psychological Testing (American Educational Research Association, American Psychological Association, &

National Council on Measurement in Education, 2014) and more specific recommendations with regard to testing from the Ethical Principals of Psychologists and Code of Conduct and any specialty guidelines promulgated by the American Psychological Association in the specific area. Finally, the evaluator should be aware of the similarity between the evaluee and those that comprise the normative group from any testing measure used. If there are substantial differences, the evaluator should choose an alternative measure or make the difference and how this may affect conclusions known in the body of the assessment report.

Collateral Records

Records from prior mental health treatments are often essential in assessing the longitudinal mental status of the evaluee. Medical records for physical conditions are often important for a global understanding of the evaluee, and also may provide confirmatory or disconfirmatory information to that provided by the evaluee in the clinical interview. School records can provide information with regard to intellectual, academic, and interpersonal functioning.

Collateral Personal Contacts

Interviews of a family member, significant other, work associate, mental health provider, or caretaker will often provide important adjunctive information. The evaluator must be sure to appropriately inform the collateral contact of the limits of confidentiality.

There may be other appropriate sources of information to be gathered depending on the unique nature of a given evaluation case.

GROWTH AND SUCCESS

As you gain experience and confidence in your evaluation and report writing skills you will gradually become thorough as well as efficient. Indeed, these are not oxymoronic concepts in the case of an assessment-based practice. You will learn to gather, organize, and express essential information, while knowing what information need not be gathered or included. You will doubtless encounter many reports in your information gathering process that have sacrificed thoroughness for efficiency, quality for profit. This will not be you. Your reports will be shining stars in what at times seems a sea of mediocrity. You will be a beacon of honesty and objectivity in a fog of partiality. Word will spread and your services will be sought after by an increasing number of referral sources.

As demand for your services increases, you will likely be faced with three choices. First, you can continue to accept more work and try to further increase your efficiency and increase your hours, perhaps working weekends, evenings, and rising earlier in the morning. This strategy will likely not only exhaust you and lead to burnout, but be unsustainable over time and become impossible as referrals continue to increase.

The second option, and that chosen by most evaluators, is to simply turn down the additional work. These evaluators simply inform the referral source that they are unable to take another case at this time, or at best may book an evaluation several months out. Most referral sources tend to be relatively displeased with the prospect of not receiving a report for several months and so eventually this strategy simply results in turning down referrals.

The third option is to hire employees or contractors who can work for the practice and allow for continued growth. Prior to taking such a step, you will want to decide whether becoming a manager and administrator in addition to a clinician is something for which you have the interest and skills. While most can develop the necessary skills to grow a business in this manner, most clinicians with whom I have met simply lack the interest, which is why they generally choose the option of turning down additional business. Should you choose to bring on other clinicians into your practice, you will need to resolve to spend a considerable portion of time engaging in administrative, management, and supervisory duties. You will very likely require the services of an office manager to assist with scheduling, billing, and general client contact, as this will likely become unwieldly for you if you are also engaging in assessment-based work yourself.

Employees are what the Internal Revenue Service (IRS) refers to as W-2 workers, and are generally provided a salary, potentially benefits, and are expected to generally follow your instructions with regard to what work they will do and how they will do it. Contractors, on the other hand, are referred to by the IRS as 1099 workers, and tend to be more independent, choosing for themselves what work they wish to do, and often being provided a percentage of the income generated. Whether you choose to bring on contractors or hire employees will depend on the nature of your referrals, your practice, and your preferred style of conducting business. Further discussions of this matter with an accountant, attorney, or trusted colleagues may be helpful.

Regardless of which you choose, significant administration and oversight will be necessary. Even if you bring on fully licensed independent individuals, nonetheless, their work product will represent your practice, so you must keep a close eye on the quality and efficiency of the work. It is simply not practical in most cases for the owner of a practice to review every report that is submitted to a referral source, but reviewing a random sample on a regular basis from each clinician in the practice is likely time well spent. You may find that some clinicians will require further supervision, have a lower level of skill than you believed them to have at the time of hire, or sadly, simply will not put in the same level of effort working for your practice that they would when performing their duties independently. Similarly, you or your office manager will likely want to keep a close eye to ensure that reports are submitted in a timely fashion as required by referral sources. In general, most referral sources will remain referral sources if they are provided a quality product submitted in a timely fashion.

You will want to make yourself available for supervision and consultation. Often new associates, be they employees or contractors, become involved in a practice because they are new to the field or less experienced in assessment. If you are carrying your own clinical load you may find this burdensome at times, but are well advised to provide such support in order to ensure the quality of your product, help your contractors/employees feel supported, and create an atmosphere of mutual assistance and collegiality. To be a helpful supervisor and consultant, you will have to remain up-to-date on the research and trends in your field, which will be important to you professionally as well.

To state the obvious, the business owner/practitioner must be aware of costs incurred versus income generated. To state the less obvious, it has been my experience that in order to maintain a practice at the highest ethical standards and quality, you will routinely find yourself eschewing opportunities for additional profits. You will be offered assessment-based cases for which no one in your practice truly has the appropriate expertise or experience. You will be offered referrals where something just does not feel right to you. Referral sources will cause a vague feeling of uneasiness and the suspicion that information is being withheld or altered in some way. At times you may seek further clarification, but on most occasions, you are best to not accept such referrals at the outset.

There will be times when you or your associates provide opinions contrary to those hoped for by a referral source. These sources may stop making referrals and that must be acceptable. There may be times when your and your associates' schedules are too full to add another case. While refusing a referral may result in less profit in the short term, in the long run, it allows you and your associates to do your best work, in an ethical fashion, for referral sources who value an honest opinion. Over time, such quality referral sources will increase and recommend you to like-minded professionals. You will find yourself in the midst of a thriving and successful mental health assessment-based practice.

REFERENCES

American Educational Research Association, American Psychological Association & National Council on Measurement in Education. (2014). *The standards for educational and psychological testing.* Washington, D.C.: American Educational Research Association.

American Psychiatric Association. (2013). *Diagnostic and statistical manual of mental disorders.* (5th Ed.). Washington, D.C.: Author.

American Psychological Association. (2010). *Ethical principles of psychologists and code of conduct.* Retrieved from http://www.apa.org/ethics/code/principles.pdf.

American Psychological Association. (2013). Specialty guidelines for forensic psychology. *American Psychologist, 68*(1), 7–19.

American Psychological Association. (2015). Medicare's shrinking psychologist reimbursement rates. Retrieved on 7/27/2015 from http://www.apapracticecentral.org/advocacy/state/leadership/medicare-payment.aspx.

Archer, R.P., Buffington-Vollum, J.K., Stredney, R.V., & Handel, R.W. (2006). A survey of psychological test use patterns among forensic psychologists. *Journal of Personality Assessment, 87*(1), 84–94.

Bow, J.N., Gould, J.W., Flens, J.R., & Greenhut, D. (2006). Testing in child custody evaluations–selection, usage, and daubert admissibility: A survey of psychologists. *Journal of Forensic Psychology Practice, 6*(2), 17–38.

Buros Center. (2014). *Buros Mental Measurements Yearbook.* (19th Ed.). Lincoln, NE: University of Nebraska Press.

Daubert v. Merrell Dow Pharmaceuticals, Inc., 509 U.S. 579 (1993).

DeRubeis, R.J., Siegle, G.J., & Hollon, S.D. (2008). Cognitive therapy vs. medications or depression: Treatment outcomes and neural mechanisms. *National Review of Neuroscience, 9*(10), 788–796.

Grove, W.M. & Lloyd, M. (2006). Meehl's contribution to clinical versus statistical prediction. *Journal of Abnormal Psychology, 115*(2), 192–194.

Heilbrun, K., Grisso, T., & Goldstein, A. (2009). *Foundations of forensic mental health assessment.* New York, NY: Oxford University Press.

Herz, G.I. (2009). Reimbursement for psychologists' services: Trends, impact on access to psychologists, and solutions. Unpublished manuscript.

McCarthy-Jones, S. & Resnick P.J. (2014). Listening to voices: The use of phenomenology to differentiate malingered from genuine auditory verbal hallucinations. *International Journal of Law and Psychiatry, 37,* 183–189.

Packer, I.K. (2009). *Evaluation of criminal responsibility: Best practices in forensic mental health assessment.* New York, NY: Oxford University Press.

Rogers, R. (ed.). (2008). *Clinical assessment of deception and malingering,* (3rd Ed.). New York, NY: The Guilford Press.

Rabin, L.A., Barr, W.A., & Burton, L.A. (2005). Assessment practices of clinical neuropsychologists in the United States and Canada: A survey of INS, NAN, and APA Division 40 members. *Archives of Clinical Neuropsychology 20*(1), 33–65.

Zusman, J., & Simon, J. (1983). Differences in repeated psychiatric examinations of litigants to a lawsuit. *American Journal of Psychiatry, 140*(10), 1300–1304.

Chapter 4

Therapist as Manager

Supervising Nonclinical Staff and Tasks

Jennifer M. Ossege and Ted Ossege

As mental health professionals, we spend a great deal of time mastering clinical skills and developing a knowledge base regarding client care, while also staying current on our own professional development; however, most of us have not received specialized training on how to manage the other aspects of practice development. As brilliant as one might be as a clinician, a clinical practice also depends on the proper management of finances, resources, and people to be successful. Since most clinicians did not also obtain a business degree as part of their graduate careers, this can be a difficult terrain to navigate and can present a challenge for many professionals in private practice.

Without the proper training or preparation for practice management, many clinicians bury themselves in clinical work and (often without realizing it) neglect important areas of their businesses. Many tell themselves, "If I can just see more clients and stay busy with billable hours, my practice will be successful." Essentially, they put their heads in the sand to avoid some of the tasks of practice management that may feel less comfortable, and definitely less familiar, than the clinical work. After all, we spent all of those years in graduate school preparing for and working toward seeing clients. Does being a great clinician automatically mean you will also be a great business manager? These skills do not automatically translate from one domain to the next, so it is important to thoughtfully consider what is involved in the management and nonclinical end of having a private practice. It is not for everyone. Running a business cannot be an afterthought, particularly if you want your practice to be successful and sustainable over time.

In this chapter, we will walk you through several considerations for managing nonclinical staff and administrative tasks. From recruiting and hiring staff and other professionals to setting up policies and procedures, it is vital to consider nonclinical staff needs, the procedures that you will need to put in place for your practice, and the nonclinical tasks that you must devote some time to in order to run your practice effectively.

THE FACE OF THE PRACTICE: SUPPORT STAFF

Whether you already have a practice and you are looking to improve it, or if you are starting fresh, it is important to consider your support staff as the face of your practice. These are the individuals that first interact with your clients (or potential clients) and often it is the support staff that others will base their initial impressions upon.

Have you viewed your practice from a new client's perspective? If you have not done so recently, you should try it. It can give you a fresh look at the experience of the consumer and help you look at what is working, as well as what could be working better. Our goal in developing our group private practice is to always step back and put ourselves in the shoes of our clients, in order to consider what we would like (or just as importantly, what we would not like) in seeking professional services. Let's consider a new client's first stages of interaction with the practice.

The client makes an initial call to inquire about services and set up an appointment with a mental health provider. What is their first impression? Are they greeted by a phone that rings and rings with no answer? Are they tossed into a voicemail system for someone to return a call to them at a later time? Or are they warmly greeted by a member of the practice support team? If you were in their shoes, which sounds best to you?

Many practices opt to have a voicemail or answering service in place of a live person answering the phone. It is understandable why this happens—hiring an employee to answer the phone can be a significant overhead expense. But we will argue that it's expensive to *not* have a support staff answering your calls. You cannot possibly know how many missed new clients simply do not leave messages on your voicemail systems and opt to go to another practice where they can talk to a person and get their questions answered right away.

Consider the client's perspective at this particular time when they make the decision to seek mental health services. Once they decide to contact a provider, it may take them days or weeks to work up the nerve to make the call to set up the initial appointment. They often put it off until there is a situation that arises that no longer lets them ignore the issue. Many do not know what to expect from a mental health provider. It can be anxiety-producing—many people are uncertain how to navigate the mental health and insurance systems, they may be intimidated and unsure about seeking mental health services in the first place, and they might even be reluctant to leave a message on a voice mail, not knowing who will be on the other end, or when their call will be returned. Some of our clients have told us that they kept calling practices until someone actually answered the phone.

In contrast, when they call an office answered by a friendly, helpful person, they can get their questions answered, an appointment scheduled, and can feel that their needs are already being met. Many of our clients report feeling relief after talking to someone at the practice who can reassure them about the process and help establish their expectations. It boosts their confidence in the practice, and thus they are off to a good start when they have their first session with the clinician.

In our practice, our goal is to have every call answered by a live support team member because we believe that the therapy process begins with this first contact. In reality, it is not always possible to meet this goal perfectly, especially when there is a high call volume, or we are short staffed due to illness. However, to help prevent missed calls, we opted for a voicemail system with the capacity to connect our three office locations with one phone system, so that support staff at each office can field the call, retrieve messages, etc. In addition we have established an option for callers to go into a call holding loop, where they can wait for the next available staff to talk to or, if they prefer to not remain on hold, they can choose to leave a message at any time. This allows options and flexibility for the client to decide what they want to do in the situation.

In essence, this initial phone contact is the first impression that the client has about you and your practice. As it is often stated, you get one chance at making a first impression, as it tends to linger. This first impression is why it is important to make sure that you hire the right person for this position. Having a warm, kind, and compassionate person interact with your prospective clients and represent your practice well is essential to getting off on the right foot. Imagine the difference it makes when you contact a business for services and the person answering the phone is rude, abrupt, or unwelcoming. It can change your impressions about that business and may make you reconsider whether you want to interact with them. Why take that chance with your practice? This is such an important factor that is often overlooked, and one that we believe is crucial to developing a thriving private practice.

When hiring the right individual (or individuals), consider what specifically you are looking for to fill this capacity. Qualities that you may want to look for when hiring support staff for your practice include friendliness, dependability, and compassion (but with good boundaries), as well as initiative, efficiency, professionalism, and good computer skills.

Support staff who will be answering phone calls from clients, welcoming clients as they enter the office, collecting payments, and helping clients schedule appointments, are an important part of the image of the practice. In our practice, many of our clients enjoy these interactions with the support staff and it enhances their experience within the practice. While it is a significant expense to hire support staff, we would argue that it is one of the best places you can spend your money. After all, everything the support staff does is one less task that you will need to do yourself. It increases overall efficiency. Your staff can answer a phone call and easily focus the call on the task at hand, whereas when a clinician returns a phone call, it is difficult to not get pulled into clinical issues that are more appropriately addressed in the therapy office (easily turning a 2 minute phone call into a 20-minute call). Hiring support staff can save you time, and free you up to see more clients. This makes your practice more efficient and makes for a better experience for your clients and for you.

WHAT OFFICE SUPPORT STAFF DO I NEED?

Whether you have a solo practice or a group practice, or you simply share office space with other clinicians, there are some basic needs you have: answering phones, scheduling appointments, managing billing, processing payments, etc. Some of these tasks can be outsourced, but you may want to know the facts before making this decision so that you don't end up paying more money than is necessary.

Administrative or Support Staff

As we discussed above, having an administrative or support staff can greatly increase your efficiency as a clinician and also enhance the client's experience. As practice owners, we have found that these staff members are invaluable—particularly as our practice grows. We are able to better focus on clients that we see and use all of the session time on important issues, rather than spending the last few minutes scheduling the next appointment (which, if you are not careful, can spill into the next scheduled therapy appointment time). There are many phone calls that office staff are able to respond to, so we have fewer phone calls to return during breaks or at the end of the day. In fact, before starting our own practice, we worked for a practice where the standard was for clients to leave voicemails for the clinician and the clinician would have to return these calls. We would spend a significant amount of time each day addressing these calls, often during our lunch breaks or at the end of a long day. This extra strain increases the chances for burnout, and makes the day less enjoyable. In starting our practice, we knew that hiring high-quality administrative staff was an important priority to us, but we were pleasantly surprised to see how much time we regained by not having nearly as many calls to return at the end of a busy day. Now, when a client cancels an appointment for the same day, our support staff is often able to fill the appointment time with another client from the waiting list before we even know that there was a cancellation (without an office staff member taking care of this, the appointment would be unfilled and therefore would result in lost income). This helps us be more efficient and be better able to serve clients and to focus on the clinical work with our clients.

Office Manager

Depending on the size and needs of your practice, you may or may not find that hiring an office manager, in addition to the other support staff positions, is needed. The role of an office manager is to oversee the processes of the support staff team. Generally, this includes arranging for scheduling, breaks, time off, etc., as well as providing supervision and support for staff, in addition to hiring new support staff and addressing any problems that arise. This individual can serve as a liaison between the clinicians, the clients, the staff, and the practice owners. In essence, the office manager helps ensure that things are running smoothly. As practice owners, we have found that having a direct line connection and regular meetings with the office manager can help keep us informed about how things are functioning. A good office manager will let the practice owners know when things are going well, but will also alert them to potential problems before they happen so they can be prevented.

Billing Manager

Have you thought about how you will collect and process your income? If you will be accepting insurance reimbursement, do you plan to bill insurance companies yourself or outsource this with a billing company? How will you handle late cancellation fees? What is your process for following up on outstanding bills or denied insurance claims?

This is one of the most important aspects of keeping your practice financially afloat. Unfortunately, it is also one of the areas that clinicians often feel unprepared to manage. Depending on the size of your practice (and the volume of claims), you may choose to manage billing on your own, outsource the practice billing tasks, or hire a billing manager within your office. We will discuss each of these options below.

1. **Managing your own billing:** Some clinicians do not want to cut into their profits in order to hire someone to manage the billing. If you are very business oriented and are willing to dedicate a sizeable portion of your time to this task, you may opt to go this route. Or if your practice does not involve any third-party payers (such as insurance companies) and you can require (and collect) all payments at the time of service, this may not be too difficult to do. However, this is more and more a rarity within a clinical practice. Also, clinicians often feel uncomfortable addressing issues of payment (or find that addressing money issues can conflict with clinical work), and this can interfere with our ability to collect payments for services rendered, and can therefore result in lost income. If you accept managed care/insurance payments, you will have to learn how to verify benefits, check deductibles, how to file electronic claims (as this is how most are processed now), proper use of Current Procedural Terminology (CPT) Codes, and logistics related to billing tasks. You will also have to learn how to follow up on denied claims, as this is unfortunately not uncommon with many insurance companies. When everything is set up correctly, however, the percentage of denied claims is really quite low. Years ago, there were times when we would swear there was a percentage of claims that were simply denied arbitrarily, but thankfully these incidents seem to occur less frequently in general. If you take the time to learn these processes and have the time to devote to this nonclinical task, you can manage your own billing. Actually submitting electronic claims to insurance companies and posting payments is not time consuming with adequate software; however, following up on denied claims can be quite time consuming. This may work for solo practitioners who only have to deal with billing issues related to their own clients. We have worked for practices that simply never followed up on denied claims. They attempted to make up for it in volume, and somehow kept plugging along, but imagine how much lost income was left out there. When you add more clinicians into the practice, billing processes can eat up a greater amount of time and can significantly cut into your billable hours.
2. **Outsourcing billing:** Another option is to outsource the task of billing through an outside service. These external billers typically charge a percentage ranging from 5 to 7 percent. The amount charged is a fixed percentage of what is collected, therefore there is some containment of the cost (as a percentage of your overhead); however, keep in mind this is on the amount collected, not billed. If you go this route, be sure to check what the collection rate is for

the outsourced billing services. You may even want to get references from other professionals who use their services to find out about what their experiences have been like, any problems they have encountered, and the collection rate that they have experienced from using the service. Do not hesitate to do your research and ask the questions that you need to ask—your income depends on it!

3. **Hiring a billing manager:** Having a billing manager within your office—a staff person specifically in charge of collecting payments from insurance companies and sending bills for outstanding accounts—can improve the efficiency (and income) of your practice. Our billing manager is like gold! She has a very high collection rate and takes pride in collecting fees that might otherwise be lost. Having a billing manager on site also allows us to keep track of and address billing issues in house and respond to client questions more efficiently. A billing manager will likely be paid on an hourly or salary basis (rather than a percentage of collections); therefore if your practice is small, this individual may also take care of tasks related to managing the front desk (answering calls, checking clients in as they arrive, etc.). As your practice grows, it will probably be necessary to have this position dedicated to the task of billing and collecting fees. In our practice, we have done this both ways. When our practice was small and just beginning, with only three or four clinicians, we were able to have one "manager" who could effectively do all of these office tasks. However, as the practice grew, we found the need to adjust the responsibilities and have a dedicated billing manager. Having a specialty billing manager also eases the process for clients who have questions about billing since they can address questions directly, and clients know who to talk to in order to resolve any issues they may be having.

HOW TO HIRE THE RIGHT PEOPLE FOR YOUR PRACTICE

Once you determine what your practice needs are, your task is to be sure that you get the right people in the right positions. Keep in mind that your needs will change as your practice changes and grows. For example, we started off with one support staff/office manager, who was in charge of most of the nonclinical work, from answering phone calls to collecting billing for the practice. At first it was just the two of us providing clinical services, so the office manager was able to meet our needs alone. Gradually, as we added providers, we also added support staff who were able to help with the needs of the practice. As our practice expanded into three office locations and multiple clinicians, our needs changed, and we now have several support staff members, an office manager and a billing manager. It has been helpful to have flexibility and the ability to reassess our needs in the process of transitioning our practice to a much larger business.

It is crucial to find the right people. This cannot be overstated. As we have discussed, the support staff will be the "face" of your practice to your clients. New or prospective clients that have a good experience with the support staff will feel comfortable and more prepared to engage in productive therapy, while those who have a negative interaction with the support staff may go elsewhere for services, or may not engage in therapy at all. Take the time to find the right people—it is one of the best things you can do to prepare your practice for success.

We have learned from experience that rushing the process is often regrettable. Unfortunately, we have learned some of these lessons the hard way. On one occasion, we hired an individual for a support position who we wanted to be a good fit for the practice. We overlooked some signs that suggested the person might struggle to keep up with the fast-paced nature of our practice. Her technical skills were a bit shaky, and she became overwhelmed trying to learn the practice software. After only a week of employment, she abruptly quit the job, leaving us in a pinch, and we had to scramble to cover our needs. We learned that it is better to take your time and get the right person for the job, rather than rushing the process because you are anxious to fill an empty position.

Finding individuals who have experience in the mental health field is helpful, but not critical. In fact, we suggest that it is much more important to get the right people who have skill sets that transfer to this line of work. There are some personal qualities that can't be taught on the job. For example, having support staff who are organized, bright, articulate, responsible, warm and friendly, and able to set good boundaries is important. If the individual has these foundational skills and abilities, then you can teach the tasks that are specific to your practice or field. Skills can transfer to new job responsibilities, but it is difficult (and often not effective) to try to change someone's personal attributes to fit a job description.

What to Look For in a Candidate

Most clinicians have not had courses in human resources or lessons on how to hire people, so this task often feels as if we are out of our comfort zone. There are lots of resources, books, articles, and workshops available to develop these skills. However, this can be time consuming, since hopefully you will not have to hire new support staff very often. In the best case, you will hire a new staff person because your practice is thriving and growing, adding to the current staff that you have. This is easier, because the new staff can work alongside the more experienced staff to learn the ropes of how the practice operates. However, in some cases you may have to hire someone to replace another employee who has left the practice for various reasons. This can sometimes leave you shorthanded, with little time to fill the gap. In this case, you may be tempted to hire someone quickly to fill the void in your eagerness to get your practice operating smoothly once again. We would caution you about moving too fast without fully vetting the new hire. As we mentioned earlier, having the wrong person in the job can be detrimental and difficult to recover from, so you want to be sure to go through the steps to make sure that you are bringing the right people on board. This may mean that you (as the practice owner) have to temporarily jump in to help with tasks that might not otherwise get accomplished in order to maintain the professionalism of your practice.

The prospect of hiring nonclinical staff can seem overwhelming to many practice owners. While we may clearly know what to ask other clinicians who may be interested in joining our practice, we are hiring nonclinical staff for a different purpose and for different tasks. It is important to remember that as clinicians, we tend to have the skillset to determine one's interpersonal skills, which makes us well suited for this task. Knowing what you are looking for—and not choosing to overlook or explain away the red flags that you may see—is an important part of the task. For example, if you really like the individual in an interview, but notice several typos and errors in their email correspondence (or worse, they do not know how to email you their resume), you can tell that their attention to detail or their technical skills may not be up to your standards. We once had a prospective employee show up 30 minutes late to the interview because she "lost track of time." While she gets points for honesty, as opposed to making up a reason having to do with traffic or a flat tire, that tardiness (especially on an interview) is a red flag not to be ignored, and she was sent away by our office manager without even an interview. Our office manager politely stated that this position requires dependability and timeliness. Although it can be difficult to turn away an otherwise viable candidate, the chances that person would have excelled in the areas of the job we needed her for were slim.

Be sure to consider the tasks that you are wanting someone to fill in the job description. If you are having to chase them down to respond to your phone calls or emails, this is not a good sign. If they are not responding to you promptly during the interview process, what makes you think this would improve once they have the job? Do you want that person to be able to work with technology and respond to client emails? Probably so. If the interviewee is already showing you some deficits in this area, pay attention to this, no matter how likeable they may be when you talk with them. In the interview process, you are likely seeing their best effort, so do not overlook key errors that provide insight into what the individual is likely to bring to their work.

How to Recruit

One of the easiest and least expensive ways to recruit new staff is to let your professional network know that you are looking for someone. Current support staff may know people who are well-suited for the job and those whom they would enjoy working with in the practice. In fact, this has been our primary way of recruiting new staff in our practice. However, you have to be aware of potential issues that may arise if the new hire does not work out for some reason. How would your current staff handle this? You should anticipate what this might mean for your practice and for your staff in advance and avoid any hiring decisions which might make it difficult to manage the staff that you have. Before hiring a friend or acquaintance of an existing staff member, you should have conversations with that staff member about your concerns and discuss potential outcomes in case things do not go as planned.

Once you have exhausted this option, and still do not have the right candidate, you may want to take out an advertisement in your local media. Find out where people who are looking for jobs seek this information in your community, which might be online, in a community paper, etc. One such option can be posting an ad on Craigslist. We recently hired someone from this resource. Out of many respondents to our Craigslist ad, five were considered viable candidates and offered an interview, although two were then quickly weeded out. Be prepared that using general advertisements will likely result in many applicants who are clearly not a good fit, but if you are patient and able to sort through these applicants, it can be a helpful and inexpensive resource to reach potential candidates. Our eventual new hire was a great fit for our office and had a skill set that could transfer to our practice setting.

If you find yourself in a time-sensitive situation, you may consider hiring a temporary office staffing service. If you find someone that you want to permanently employ, there is often an associated cost, so you should find out all of these details in advance.

Don't Settle or Rush to Hire

Although you may feel pressure to quickly fill an open support staff position, we want to caution you to be sure to do your due diligence. Take the time to properly interview, check references, and be sure that the individual you are hiring will be a good fit for your practice. Hiring the wrong person can be expensive and aggravating. It can be a difficult mistake to fix. For this reason, we suggest when hiring support staff that you consider building in a probationary period of about 3 months before determining whether the support staff member is a good fit for the permanent position. At the end of the probationary period you can sit down with the individual and determine if the person is a good fit for you and the practice. Be sure to check out the employment laws in your state to remain compliant.

DEVELOPING POLICIES AND PROCEDURES

As a solo practice, clearly written policies and procedures are not likely necessary, unless you plan to add employees in the future and want to have guidelines for how things will work. Other practice owners might think this is completely unnecessary—that is, until you find that you need the documentation to support a termination, or need guidance to maintain consistency. Basically, if you have employees or contractors, clinicians and/or support staff, it is a good idea to clearly define the expectations of the practice. This helps to ensure that everyone is on the same page. You can develop one Policy and Procedure Manual, or have two separate manuals, whichever works best for your practice. After you disseminate the manuals to your employees, it is important to get them to sign off on a form stating that they have received and reviewed the manual. This will help avoid the "I didn't know…" excuse when a policy is violated, and can help you hold people accountable.

Policy Manual

A policy manual can be simple, but it should be clear. Essentially, a policy manual should describe the employment or contractor relationship as well as the culture, or expectations, of the practice. You should carefully consider what your expectations and legal responsibilities are as you create the policy manual. Having an attorney review the manual is suggested in order to ensure that the manual meets legal criteria in case there is conflict between an employee and yourself, as the practice owner. Below is a list of some of the practice policies that you may want to consider including in your Policy Manual (although the list is not exhaustive):

- Sexual harassment and other legal policies
- Drug/alcohol policy
- Employee classifications and work hours
- Inclement weather and emergency policy

- Personal appearance expectations
- Expectations of employees
- Expectations of employers
- Benefits for professional and nonclinical staff
- Leave of absence policies
- Policy on outside employment
- Confidentiality policy
- Termination policy

Procedure Manual

A Procedure Manual deals more with the operational end of the practice. It is a helpful tool to have when training new staff or holding current staff accountable to the procedures that have been established. Be sure to update your Procedure Manual regularly to reflect changes as they occur. If it is outdated, it will not be used. A list of suggested procedures is below (but may vary widely depending on your practice operations):

- Regular work hours
- Job descriptions
- Procedures for handling intakes and other processes related to client care
- Procedures for psychological evaluations or other assessments
- Standards of conduct
- Disciplinary action process and appeals process
- Termination

ESTABLISHING OTHER PROFESSIONAL RELATIONSHIPS

As you consider developing your practice, in addition to hiring clinical staff and support or administrative staff within the practice itself, it is likely you will want to make several professional connections to help you navigate other areas of your business.

Attorneys

While you may not have ongoing needs that require the attention of an attorney, there are some areas in which consulting with an attorney can be particularly helpful, especially when you are just starting out. Of course, it can also be advantageous to have an attorney on retainer, or at least available for consultation, in case any legal issues arise, such as guidance on how to handle subpoenas or how to reduce risk and liability to your practice.

When you are forming your practice, consulting with an attorney can be essential, particularly in knowing what legal hoops you need to go through to avoid any problems and ensure that your practice is legally sound. Your attorney can help guide you with obtaining a business license, establishing your Articles of Incorporation, or in handling other documents needed for the type of business that you are establishing.

It is also a good idea (even if somewhat morbid) to set up a plan for what would happen to your practice in the case of your death or incapacity. This can be formalized in a will, so that in the case of your death it will be clear what your wishes are as to who might take over your clinical cases and how your practice affairs would be run, as well as if the practice changes hands or is shut down upon your death. Nobody wants to think about this possibility, but it is important to get something established and formalized so that there is a plan in place. Then you can go about running and enjoying your clinical practice knowing that contingencies are already established.

Accountants

Maybe you are great with numbers and feel confident with filing taxes for yourself and your practice. If so, good for you! However, the reality is that most of us rely on experts to help us file our taxes, and to advise us on issues related to financial aspects of running our businesses. There are many issues that can arise and details to keep track of when it comes to items such as taxes and payroll, and it likely is not worth your time to try and stay ahead of it all. If you are one of the majority who need a little help in this area, be sure to interview some accountants, or ask colleagues about the accounting firms they use, and gather recommendations. It can be helpful to find out whether the accountant has dealt with other small businesses like your practice before you hire them. It is one of those areas where a small expense now can save some major expenses in the future.

Your ongoing needs will differ widely, depending on the scale and size of your practice. If you are a solo practitioner with no employees, filing your taxes will not be as complicated as a larger practice that employs many clinicians and support staff. Whether you have set your business up as a corporation or a professional limited liability company (PLLC or LLC) will determine whether you need to file quarterly estimated taxes or just an annual return.

There are many bookkeeping software programs on the market that are user friendly and relatively inexpensive. Many of us running a practice can manage the day-to-day bookkeeping tasks fairly easily without it being too burdensome. You will likely not have to outsource this task, particularly if your accountant can show you how to utilize the program from the beginning. However, if managing finances is not for you, it can be a task that you can delegate to a third party. However, a cautionary note is to always be aware of the finances of your business so that you can continue to keep expenses and costs in check and so that you are not taken advantage of. We have a colleague who allowed the office manager of his practice to run the finances. He was unaware of money going in and out of his practice, and relied on this staff person to provide him with money for daily living expenses. Unfortunately, he learned the hard way that while he had trusted this employee implicitly, she had taken advantage of this trust and embezzled money from the practice. This was a person whom he had relied on in the past to care for his children. He never dreamed this staff person would be capable of this action. Since he was not aware of the details of the finances or how his cash flow worked, it took years for this to come to light. If you outsource your bookkeeping tasks to an employee or another individual, be sure to remain aware of where the stream of money is going and be able to take over this task at any point if the need arises.

Prior to beginning our practice, we did not have bookkeeping experience (that is, outside of balancing our personal checkbooks). Aside from a couple of accounting classes in college and graduate school, we did not know much about keeping track of financials and found this a bit intimidating. Our accounting firm recommended a software program and spent some time up front teaching us how to use it properly. Initially, our bookkeeping was fairly simple, with only one office location and the two of us practicing as owners (thus no employees). However, our practice quickly grew and we added support staff and other clinicians, which made our bookkeeping tasks a bit more complex as well. Before we knew it, our annual collections (as a practice) were over $800,000. As you can imagine, when collections are higher, the payroll for employees are higher and the expenses are higher, therefore the bookkeeping tasks became busier with increased volume.

Payroll Specialists

Whether or not you have a need for using a payroll specialist will depend on whether you have employees. If you are a solo practice with no employees, this does not pertain to you. However, if you have employees (rather than contractors) you may want to consider hiring a payroll company to manage your payroll for you. Yes, this is another overhead expense, but payroll calculations can be complex. In fact, when we started our practice, our accountant recommended that we use a payroll specialist because the penalties are high if you make mistakes in calculating payroll taxes.

Actually, even though he is a CPA and his accounting firm is full of competent accountants, his practice also uses a payroll specialist service!

Having a payroll specialist or payroll company is not very time intensive or difficult on the practice management end. It also is not very expensive and is well worth the small amount it will cost. You can establish the frequency of your pay periods and you will have regular days in which you need to process your payroll by. In doing this you will enter the hours worked (for hourly employees) or the dollar amount to be paid (for clinical staff) and the payroll amounts will be calculated. The payroll company often sets up direct deposits to make payroll easier for employees and they file the taxes on behalf of your practice. They also take care of all the quarterly taxes that many cities and municipalities require. It is a real headache to try and keep track of all these varying deadlines, laws, tax rates, etc. on your own. Records are all available online, and when we recently had a routine audit by the state, all records were easily available, and the audit went very smoothly. Preparing for the audit was simply a matter of downloading records from the payroll company's website, and literally, that is all we had to do, reducing the anxiety associated with the audit.

Insurance Agent/Broker

Many small practices cannot afford to pay health insurance benefits for their employees, although this does not mean that you cannot help your employees ensure that they have the health insurance coverage they need. Establishing a relationship with an insurance agent/broker can be a step toward making the process easier for your employees. They can contact the insurance agent/broker individually and work through finding a plan that works for them.

Additionally, there are some companies that offer supplemental insurance policies for employees, with little cost to your practice beyond minimal fees to establish the account.

Retirement Specialist

Another perk that you can establish for interested employees (with minimal startup costs) is a retirement account. Even if you cannot (or choose to not) contribute to or match the retirement funds, it can still be a valuable service for the clinicians working in your practice. There are many rules and regulations about what type of account you can set up based on whether you will contribute to it, whether you will participate in it yourself, etc. Therefore, it is helpful to consult with a retirement specialist about how to establish the proper accounts and how this can work for you and your practice.

WORKING ON YOUR BUSINESS WHILE WORKING IN YOUR BUSINESS

Whether you are a solo practitioner or an employer, chances are that you will have a busy clinical caseload to help generate revenue. This is important in order to pay your bills and to provide the type of satisfaction that you have come to expect as a mental health professional. But what about the other things that do not result in direct billing? What about the marketing of your practice or developing and maintaining good referral streams? What about the financial management and the practice management tasks? How can you successfully manage these tasks while you are seeing a full caseload of clients?

One of the big shifts from working for an agency or for another practice to being the boss yourself is that you have to spend a great deal of time working *on* your business, at the same time as you are working *in* your business. Essentially, it is important as a practice manager to reduce your caseload to accommodate the other necessary tasks of running a practice. For some people, this is a welcome change of pace and allows them to utilize a different set of skills. For others, it can simply be overwhelming. You need to make sure that you are willing to engage in hours of practice management tasks on a regular basis, and to oversee the actions of others whom you have hired, if you want to run a practice. If this is not for you, that's okay. You may find it is more your style to join a group practice where someone else takes care of these tasks for you, allowing you to focus on your clinical caseload.

You should carefully consider the questions below before choosing to open your own practice:

- Which tasks do you plan to take care of yourself and which would you prefer to outsource?
- Are you going to hire support staff or do you plan to answer phones, schedule, and return calls yourself?
- Do you plan to do your own bookkeeping or outsource this to an employee or other professional?
- Who will do the billing for your practice? Do you plan to do it yourself, hire a billing manager (who will require some supervision), or do you plan to outsource this task?
- Are you going to calculate payroll yourself, hire an accountant to do it, or go with a payroll company? If you use a payroll company, how much time will it take to enter payroll information each time?
- When will you have time to hire new staff or clinicians, update policy and procedural manuals, etc.?

- How will you regularly meet with your office manager and billing manager to ensure that things are running smoothly?

Each of these tasks takes time, and since there are a finite number of hours in the day (and only a certain amount of those hours you are willing to dedicate to your work), each task will inevitably take away from your clinical hours. While you may have been able to see 40 clients a week when you worked for another practice where someone else took care of these tasks, your clinical hours may be reduced to 25 or 30, depending on the tasks you take on. You will need to consider this reduction in your clinical hours when you are calculating the costs associated with outsourcing various jobs. Also, you should determine whether it appeals to you to have these tasks built into your work week, or whether you feel that it would pull you away from your "real" work. In running a practice, your "real" work will be redefined beyond your clinical cases. It will be necessary to engage in tasks that keep your practice running (e.g., generating referrals to the practice, managing the billing and financial end of things, overseeing the operations of the practice, filling support staff and clinical staff positions, etc.).

One of the advantages we enjoyed in starting our practice was that one of us was very good at managing people, finances, and administrative activities, and the other was skilled in technology, software, and computers. Some of the duties were then able to be divided based on our areas of interest, ability, and expertise. We often comment that one of the advantages of running our own practice is being able to do things requiring different parts of our brain other than we use in providing therapy, such as networking computers, budgeting office expenses, or solving insurance billing issues. We enjoy the variety of tasks that managing nonclinical staff and tasks requires.

CONCLUSION

This chapter has explored the many aspects of managing nonclinical staff and nonclinical tasks. These areas tend to be new (and perhaps intimidating) for the professional who is venturing into the world of establishing a private practice, as our training has been centered around clinical knowledge and skills development, rather than business management and accounting.

If you are just starting out in a solo or group practice, or deciding to grow your practice, it can be helpful to have a better idea of some of the decisions that you will need to make as well as the tasks involved in running a practice. Keep in mind that as a trained clinician, you have several skills which can translate into many business practices, such as human resources, management, and marketing, as well as in building relationships necessary to bring referrals into your practice.

One of the mistakes that practitioners make when starting their own practice is that they overlook the importance of running the business side of the practice. By being better informed about what is entailed in the development and maintenance of a private practice you can be sure to not neglect these important tasks. You may even find that you enjoy the new challenges that come along with establishing and sustaining a practice that thrives.

There are many wonderful aspects of managing the nonclinical aspects of your private practice! By being well informed and anticipating the needs of your practice in the short and long terms, you will be better positioned to embrace the new challenges and opportunities that you will face as a practice manager. Instead of avoiding the tasks that intimidate you, we encourage you to talk to your colleagues who are in private practice about their experiences, consult with your mentors to get help to learn the tasks that are unfamiliar to you, and be proactive in the management of your practice. By doing so, you will be able to build your practice exactly the way you want!

SUGGESTED READING

Hunt, H. (2005). *Essentials of private practice: Streamlining costs, procedures and policies for less stress.* New York, NY: W.W. Norton & Company.

Paterson, R.J. (2011). *Private practice made simple: Everything you need to know to set up and manage a successful mental health practice.* Oakland, CA: New Harbinger Publications.

Steele, D. (2012). *The million dollar private practice: Using your expertise to build a business that makes a difference.* Hoboken, NJ: John Wiley & Sons.

Stout, C.E., & Grand, L.C. (2005). *Getting started in private practice: The complete guide to building your mental health practice.* Hoboken, NJ: John Wiley & Sons.

Walfish, S. & Barnett, J.E. (2009). *Financial success in mental health practice: Essential tools and strategies for practitioners.* Washington, D.C.: American Psychological Association.

Yenney, S. & American Psychological Association Practice Directorate. (1994). *Business strategies for a caring profession: A practitioner's guidebook.* Washington, D.C.: American Psychological Association.

Chapter 5

Navigating the Digital Landscape

A Practitioner's Guide to Moving Through the Rough Terrain of the Internet and Social Media

Jami Wilder and Heather Wilder

Microsoft cofounder Bill Gates once said, "The Internet is becoming the town square for the global village of tomorrow." Advances in technology are shrinking the "global village" through increased connection. For the "village's" providers of mental healthcare, the changes in the digital landscape have altered not only the way we are hanging out the proverbial shingle, but have changed the shingle itself.

In a matter of minutes, a person can visit a zoo in China, scroll through the Yelp reviews of a restaurant, zip through the daily headlines on Twitter, and search for information about a potential therapist for marriage counseling. That same person can pull up the clinician's professional review profiles, practice website, Facebook profile, pictures of the practitioner on Google's image search, and find directions to the provider's home on Google Maps—all before she has finished her morning coffee or decided to engage services.

Since the advent and proliferation of the Internet, access to information has wildly expanded, which, in turn, is quickly reducing the barriers between people. According to the Pew Research Center, 84 percent of adults in the United States use the Internet (Perrin & Duggan, 2015). Social media sites like Facebook, Twitter, and LinkedIn report millions of daily users. Facebook reported an average of 936 million daily users in March 2015 (Facebook, 2015). In the same month, Twitter reported 302 million active users from around the globe (Twitter, 2015). LinkedIn reported that its network connects 346 million professionals worldwide (LinkedIn, 2015). Mental health practitioners are among those engaged online. For clinicians in private practice, a digital presence is a vital part of building a practice, delivering services, and connecting with current and potential clients.

Online professional activities serve as marketing and brand development for practitioners in individual and group practice. Practice websites, Facebook pages, Twitter feeds, and LinkedIn profiles allow providers to market themselves and the services they offer. In addition to websites and social media, blog posts and other online contributions provide opportunities to educate the public about specialties, practice philosophy, and areas of interest (Kolmes, 2012; Poeppleman & Blacksmith, 2014). By contributing to the digital landscape, clinicians are increasing accessibility and decreasing barriers to treatment. This may be particularly helpful to traditionally underserved populations and individuals who are hesitant to access services (Kolmes, 2012). Additionally, technological advances allow for quick, timely, and efficient communication with clients, improving service and streamlining many of the administrative tasks private practitioners face.

While the expanding technological landscape offers opportunities to reach and connect with clients, it also presents legal and ethical quagmires for private practice clinicians. The expansion of information access and shrinking barriers comes with challenges to the relationship between therapist and client. With access to an almost unlimited supply of information and to one another's digital lives, therapists and their current and potential clients are met with an intersectionality of their personal and professional worlds. This intersectionality creates ethical, legal, and clinical challenges, which are emerging at a faster pace than development of practice standards and research on the impact.

For those clinicians looking for a compass to navigate the digital landscape, some guidance can be found in emerging literature and guidelines issued by professional organizations. For example, the American Psychological Association (APA) issued *Guidelines for the Practice of Telepsychology* (American Psychological Association, 2013). Developed by the Joint Task Force for the Development of Telepsychology Guidelines for Psychologists, the primary focus of the guidelines is on the delivery of psychological care via technology. Within those aspirational guidelines, the task force highlights ethical considerations related to all telecommunication including the Internet, social media, and email. The APA is not alone in its efforts to provide some measure of guidance for its members. The *American Counselors Association Code of Ethics* also includes provisions regarding clinician activity with digital technology and social media (American Counselors Association, 2014). As professional organizations and authors are attempting to address issues presented by our digital interactions, technology is shifting at a rapid pace, making it difficult to provide specific guidelines for all possible ethical and legal challenges that might be encountered in the daily practice. This chapter provides an overview of some of the ethical and legal considerations that private practitioners may encounter. Additionally, specific recommendations are provided to assist clinicians in navigating the intersectionality of digital lives.

NAVIGATING ETHICAL AND LEGAL CONCERNS

The intersection of digital lives in Mr. Gates' metaphorical town square of the global village may be akin to life in rural or closely connected communities. The connections created by digital means are similar to ones often experienced by those therapists working in small communities and in communities where therapists share overlapping identity variables with clients, like ability status, sexual orientation, cultural backgrounds, or religious/spiritual affiliations (Kolmes, 2012; Nicholson, 2011). The nature of the information online means that therapists have access to clients in a way that is similar to running into them at the grocery store or hearing about them from a mutual acquaintance. We can see aspects of their lives that may be very separate from what they share in session, and vice versa. The bidirectionality of the digital information means clients may see aspects of our lives that we may not intend for them to see. Unintentional crossings and accidental disclosure of information by the therapist or others in the therapist's lives can occur through social media in avenues like Facebook's Friends of Friends feature.

The experience of clinicians working in small, closely connected communities illuminates some of the ethical concerns for all clinicians who have a digital presence, whether they created it or not. Issues related to privacy for both the client and the clinician, maintaining confidentiality, providing ongoing and adequate informed consent, and guarding against multiple relationships must all be considered along with the impact of digital encounters on the therapeutic relationship.

Develop Digital Competence

In considering the ethical implications of engaging with the digital landscape, practitioners must explore many of the same considerations that they would in the "real" world. Maintaining privacy and protecting confidentiality are still of utmost importance. Providing informed consent and guarding against multiple relationships with clients must still be considered. While the tenets of good, ethical practice have not changed, the landscape in which it must be conducted comes with new challenges.

First and foremost, as we engage with the digital landscape, it is important to consider the ethical obligation to provide services only within the boundaries of our clinical competence (American Psychological Association, 2010). Educating ourselves about the tools that we are utilizing to create and sustain a digital presence is as important as engaging in continuing education in areas like treatment modalities and diagnosis (American Psychological Association, 2013). The Internet, email, and social media have become important components of our business. However, they are not only necessary for business, they are also important because our clients' lives are intertwined with the digital landscape (Kolmes, 2012). For example, many clients are deeply impacted by interactions with significant others on dating sites, by cyberbullying or stalking, and by seeing the "happy" lives of others on Facebook. In an effort to help them cope with the impact, clinicians must have a working knowledge of the digital landscape and an understanding of the implications of participating in it. Nicholson (2011) noted that while we are not required to become technology experts, we do need to be informed consumers who can weigh the risks and benefits of the technology and discuss those with our clients.

Privacy Issue: You Saw Me Where?

Digitally competent providers know that the digital landscape grants readily available access to information. Providers who are active in the digital world know that with a few keystrokes on the computer or mobile device, a person's documented life is available. This presents challenges in maintaining and protecting the privacy of our clients. With a quick Google search, a provider can learn more about their clients than the clients wish to disclose. Kolmes and Taube (2014) surveyed providers about intentional and unintentional online encounters. Results of the survey showed that 28 percent of participants have experienced accidental online discovery of current client information, noting that the largest percentage of those occurred on Facebook, followed by Google, LinkedIn, shared email lists, blogs, and Twitter. The study showed a small number (3 percent) occurred on dating sites.

In regard to intentional searches, Kolmes and Taube (2014) found 48 percent of participants intentionally sought information about clients in a noncrisis situation without the client's awareness. A small percentage (8 percent) searched during moments of crises. Those who searched during noncrisis moments did so for a variety of reasons ranging from seeking general information related to treatment or verification of information shared in treatment; searching for information like police records, blog updates during hospitalization, photographs, and information about the client's relationships, to determine if the client was a member of the clinician's extended social network, or for misplaced contact information.

Harris and Kurpius (2014) studied the online behaviors of graduate students and found similar reasons for seeking out clients in the digital world. They found that participants who had more familiarity with social networking were more likely to engage in searches for client information. Eighty percent of students who searched did not obtain client consent nor did they document the search in the clinical records. They also did not consider it a breach of confidentiality. Curiosity was the most cited reason for searching. Harris and Kurpius (2014) suggested that searching for curiosity's sake could be considered unethical because it violates the right to privacy.

Clients have the right to decide how much of their lives and experiences they share with others, including with their mental healthcare providers. The proliferation of personal information on the Internet may make it incredibly difficult for clients to maintain their privacy. Some clinicians may suggest that information shared on social media sites are inherently public and, therefore, nullify the expectation of privacy. Harris and Kurpius (2014) noted that the intention of the clinician in accessing the information, and the way in which it is accessed, should be considered. They went on to say that, like a chance encounter in person with a client, stumbling upon digital information about a client is different than actively searching it out without the client's consent. The authors likened intentional searches without consent to observing clients in person without their knowledge or consent, which is unethical.

Clinicians are encouraged to consider the impact of accessing client information, intentionally or otherwise. Studies conducted about this impact showed conflicting results in regard to the clinicians' beliefs regarding how the information impacted the relationship (Kolmes & Taube, 2014). Learning details of our clients' lives that they may not have felt comfortable sharing with us may change the nature of the relationship, for the positive or negative. It may influence our interactions with them. Additionally, clinicians who learn details that are not shared in session must decide how to approach discussing the information and how that information was learned. Consider the impact of discovering that a client is still smoking when you are working on smoking cessation, or if you learn that a client is involved in a romantic relationship that you thought had ended. Learning this information may change the therapeutic focus. It may also be a time for clinicians to engage in reflection about the nature of the therapeutic relationship with the particular client and what factors may be contributing to withholding of information from the therapist. Some argue that this may help the work. But we must consider what would be the cost in terms of the client's autonomy and fundamental right to privacy (Nicholson, 2011).

Protecting client privacy extends beyond our own searches for clients. Attention to privacy concerns must also include awareness of the impact of location-based services (LBS) (Kolmes, 2012). LBS are present on many phone applications (apps) like 4Square and Twitter. The services enable apps and websites through GPS on a mobile device to determine the location of the device (and thereby the device's owner). With LBS on a device, clients may transmit their location and alert others to their participation in therapy. This may also be concerning for clients who are in danger from others in their lives, like survivors of domestic abuse. For most apps and websites, the client must "check-in," "tweet," or post something for their location to be made public. While clients may be knowingly making their private lives and location public, they may not have considered the impact of giving up privacy of the therapy space. Because of the inadvertent public disclosure of participation in therapy through LBS, it may be important to increase client awareness of potential privacy concerns.

Confidentiality: "Friends of Friends"

In addition to privacy concerns, our ethical duty to maintain client confidentiality can be particularly challenging in the digital space. Much like real-world encounters that may occur with some frequency in closely connected communities, therapists and clients may find that overlapping digital networks can make it difficult to not inadvertently reveal the nature of their relationships online. In truth, total confidentiality online cannot be guaranteed, a fact that must be discussed in the therapeutic space. From email communication to social media participation, we must acknowledge and prepare for the possibility that third parties may gain access to client-identifying information (Bradley, Hendricks, Lock, Whiting, & Parr, 2011). Baker and Bufka (2011) stated that some state licensing boards have strongly encouraged clinicians to discuss the risks of using unsecured forms of electronic communication like some email services.

In regard to social media, complications arise in several ways. First, social media sites are predicated on the notion of building social networks. One method through which that is accomplished is linking together "Friends of Friends" (in the case of Facebook) or helping you find "People You Might Know" (in the case of LinkedIn). The service may link therapists with clients if their online social networks have overlaps. Accepting those invitations to connect with clients blurs the lines of professional and personal space, allowing your clients and your loved ones to mingle online. This mingling introduces many complicating factors including the potential for disclosure of content that may violate the client's confidentiality. Additionally, providers who use their social media pages as business pages create problematic relationship connections and risk as clients can leave comments that may breach confidentiality (Anderson & Guyton, 2013). In an effort to navigate the potential overlap of personal and professional connections, practitioners may consider establishing business pages. Most social media sites allow for the creation of pages that establish and maintain professional interactions. For providers who establish business pages, it is important to discuss with clients the impact of confidentiality in engaging with the pages.

Direct engagement with the digital landscape is not the only way providers should consider confidentiality concerns. Review websites, like Yelp and Healthgrade, often create profiles for service providers and businesses without knowledge or permission. The public, including clients, can post reviews of therapists on these sites. While some of the sites offer businesses the opportunity to post a public response to any review, therapists who follow the APA ethics code cannot respond to reviews without breaking confidentiality. To do so would identify the reviewer as a client (Kolmes, 2012). For former clients posting reviews, we may have no recourse to address the situations or to respond. For current clients, we may be able to utilize the review in the therapeutic experience but cannot respond publicly.

Informed Consent: Give All the Facts

In discussing the limits of confidentiality and potential privacy concerns, clinicians will need to address the overlap of digital lives, concerns related to the transmission of information via the Internet, and ways in which technology could be influential in the therapeutic relationship. Alerting clients to unintentional and intentional exposure to online information is also important in giving the client the opportunity to provide informed consent about their participation in therapy (Lehavot, Barnett, & Powers, 2010). Informed consent must be an ongoing process in which clients are informed of changes in circumstances that will impact them and the care that they receive (American Psychological Association, 2010). Therefore, as issues arise (e.g., receiving a "Friend Request" from a client), clinicians will need to provide explanations about the how they will be navigated.

APA's Guidelines for Telepsychology (2013) suggest that clients be informed of the types of telecommunication that clinicians use in the course of treatment (e.g., email, social media, text, voicemail). Additionally, clients should be informed about the clinician's policies related to telecommunication. By establishing policies about the use of email communication, social media, practice websites, and other online interaction, therapists provide expectations and an understanding of protections for client and clinician digital spaces (see Table 5.1 for samples of social media and website policies). Informed consent discussions about digital

Table 5.1 Website and Social Media Policies—Sample Text[1]

Type of policy	*Text options*
Client endorsements	You may find a profile for [PRACTICE NAME], or our providers, on websites which invite visitors to provide a review or endorsement of our services. It should be noted that our presence on those websites is not a request for your endorsement. Many websites post listings for professionals without their knowledge or consent. Clients should be aware that they are entitled to confidentiality and that providing a review of services will reveal the nature of their relationship to their provider.
Website comments	Comments made on websites, including [PRACTICE NAME] website, will not be responded to as we have an ethical duty to protect your confidentiality. Clients should be aware that they are entitled to confidentiality and that providing a comment on a provider's website may reveal the nature of their relationship to the provider.
Internet searches	Your privacy is important to us. To maintain your privacy, [PRACTICE NAME] will not search for you or access online information about you without your consent. Any explorations conducted, even with consent, will be conducted for relevant therapeutic reasons only. Accidental discoveries of your personal digital information will be disclosed promptly.
Social media	Providers of [PRACTICE NAME] will not accept "friend requests" or invitations to connect or be linked on social media sites since this constitutes a dual relationship that can negatively impact therapeutic relationships. If shared social media connections are found to pose a potential threat to confidentiality, clients may be blocked to ensure the privacy of both therapist and client.

[1] Since ethics codes and local statutes vary, seek professional counsel for your specific needs.

technologies should also include exploration of the risks to clients of utilizing electronic methods of communication. For example, clients should be informed about the risk associated with sending personal information through nonencrypted email accounts. Beyond the discussion, clinicians should consider making policies readily available to clients by posting them on practice websites. Email policy and an informed consent statement can be included in the signature area of emails sent by the clinician (see Table 5.2 for sample email policies).

Impact on Therapeutic Relationships

Discussion and policies related to informed consent, confidentiality, and privacy also help to establish the parameters of the therapeutic relationship

Table 5.2 Email Policies—Sample Text[1]

Type of policy	*Text options*
Email signature	*Confidentiality notice:* email is not a secure form of communication and may be vulnerable to interception by an unintended party. You have received this email because you have given permission to receive unsecured communication from this provider. If you wish to remove consent for email communication, please contact [PHONE #].
Email uses	In light of the potential risks to your confidentiality, [PRACTICE NAME] asks that you use email to facilitate scheduling and do not use email to discuss personal issues.
Email response (1)	*Important note:* email messages may not be read each day so please contact us by phone if you have a time-sensitive matter to discuss. If you are having a psychological emergency, please call 911.
Email response (2)	*Important note:* email messages will be read and responded to each day between [TIME]. Please contact us by phone if you have a time-sensitive matter to discuss. If you are having a psychological emergency, please call 911.
Email signature: confidentiality	This email message is for the intended recipient(s) only as it may contain private and/or privileged information that is governed by legal protections. If you are not the intended recipient(s), please delete this message and notify the sender promptly.
Unsecured electronic communications	Due to the ease of electronic communication, many clients prefer to reach us by email or text message. Email and text messaging are not secure forms of communication and may be vulnerable to interception by an unintended party. For the convenience of our clients, it is the practice of this office to send email reminders of appointments. However, you are free to opt out of receiving all electronic communications from us.
Consent to email	I understand the potential risks of unsecured email communication and agree to receive email messages from [PRACTICE NAME] ____________________.
Opt out of email	I do not wish to be contacted by email and I opt out of appointment reminders and all electronic communication from [PRACTICE NAME] ____________________.

[1] Since ethics codes and local statutes vary, seek professional counsel for your specific needs.

within the digital space and within the real world. Access to an abundance of information, overlapping social connections, and the casual and colloquial nature of communication that occurs in the digital space can lead to the perception of blurred lines between a professional and a personal relationship. For example, email communication can often lead to misinterpretation because of the lack of nonverbal information (Bradley,

Hendricks, Lock, Whiting, & Parr, 2011). This lack of interpersonal cues in digital communication may be problematic. Colloquial text communication mechanisms, such as using emoticons and abbreviations like LOL (laugh out loud), may provide some interpersonal cues and enhance the relationship, but may also create a false sense of intimacy.

To counter the blurring of the clinical relationship that might occur through email, Bradley, Hendricks, Lock, Whiting, and Parr (2011) recommended that practitioners explain the boundaries and limitations, including how email will be used and what kind of content will be responded to (e.g., administrative tasks, scheduling, billing) and will not be responded to in email (e.g., discussing clinical issues). Practical considerations that can impact the therapeutic relationship should also be discussed and addressed in practice policies, including fees for responding to email if charged, and during what hours clients can expect responses (see Table 5.2 for sample policies).

In addition, social media encounters may have an impact on the clinical relationship. For instance, clinicians must consider the impact of accepting or ignoring requests to connect via social media by clients. Anderson and Guyson (2013) noted that requests must be considered within the context of the entire therapeutic relationship. The decision to connect may vary by client for some practitioners. If an invitation is accepted, clinicians must weigh the impact of later "unfriending" the client if problems arise. Clinicians must also consider whether connecting with clients online through social sites may constitute an ethically prohibited dual relationship. Currently, there is little definitive guidance in the literature or from professional organizations regarding whether social media connections constitute a prohibited dual relationship.

Legal Concerns: Violation of Confidentiality and Privacy

Most clinicians are aware that sharing identifying confidential information about clients without consent violates ethical principles and legal statutes. Even seemingly benign disclosures online may put practitioners at legal risk (Harris & Kurpius, 2014). Reports in the media and lawsuits in the courts are emerging following disclosures by healthcare providers who assumed that sharing some aspects of encounters with patients/clients would not violate confidentiality. For instance, a paramedic and his employer were sued following a post on the paramedic's social media site regarding care he provided to an unnamed survivor of rape (Clark, 2010).

It is important to consider how easily one might breach a client's confidentiality online. Email can be inadvertently sent to the wrong email address. Posting about your long day of client interactions may identify a client who happens to be a friend of your friend connected through social media. Responding to client posts on your business page in a way that would indicate that a professional relationship exists, essentially resulting in "outing" the person as your psychotherapy client. In such occurrences, providers are obligated to alert clients to the breach of confidentiality. The legal and ethical implications and obligations of digital confidentiality breaches necessitate action just as breaches in other ways do.

Legal statutes and regulations that are relevant to online practice concerns vary by state. For instance, some state laws include informed consent requirements for clinicians to discuss how electronic communication (e.g., emails) is stored (Baker & Bufka, 2011). Clinicians are encouraged to consult the state laws and regulations in which they practice regarding informed consent, privacy, and confidentiality statutes and guidelines.

On a federal level, practitioners should be aware of the intersection between the Health Insurance Portability and Accountability Act of 1996 (HIPAA) and digital interactions. HIPAA outlines the privacy and security standards that protect identifiable health information. It applies to providers and their business associates (e.g., insurance companies) who electronically transmit and store personal health information (PHI).

HIPAA is designed to allow for flexibility in what safeguards should be taken and does not provide specific technological requirements or practices needed to be compliant with the rules. This allows providers and practices to set and implement policies that fit the size and function of the business (Baker & Bufka, 2011). As noted by Zur (2014), providers need to consider insuring safety measures like password protection, firewalls, virus protection, and backup systems, as well as other computer-safety measures in an effort to be HIPAA compliant.

Since the inception of HIPAA, clarifying statements and guidance about email communication in particular have been provided, most recently in 2013. Zur (2014) highlighted HIPAA clarification regarding the use of unencrypted email to communicate with clients. The HIPAA clarification in 2013 allowed providers to use unencrypted email if the client fully understands the risks and agrees for information to be sent over unsecured email. The second condition is that providers have conducted and documented their own analysis of available electronic communication options, examining cost, risk, applicability to the practice, and security (Zur, 2014). If a particular option is too expensive or too cumbersome for the provider or practice, HIPAA allows for them to forgo encryption (e.g., secured email), as long as the clients are informed of the risks. In addition to discussing email policies with clients, providers can also include statements with each email that outline the dangers and limitation of sending information through email (see Table 5.2 for sample text). The primary goal is to alert clients of potential dangers and to support the autonomy of their informed choice in communication.

Protecting Your Space

While clinicians work to maintain the privacy and confidentiality of our clients, the ever-expanding access clients gain through the digital world may lead them to expect more information about us. Zur and Donner (2009) stated that the greater transparency of the Internet may require therapists to give consideration to how they understand and define self-disclosure.

Personal information, no matter how closely monitored, may leak into the professional realm without clinicians putting it there. For example, you may attend a family member's birthday party. A relative, who has no concerns for privacy, may post pictures of the party on Facebook, using the site's tagging feature to include you in the post. Tech-savvy clients or those who have some overlap with your social circle may gain access to the photos, which can disclose more information than would ever be shared within the confines of the therapeutic relationship.

Most digital information is saved in some form in perpetuity, meaning that our digital lives are forever documented and accessible. For many early-career mental health providers and student practitioners who are often considered "digital natives," a significant portion of their lives prior to becoming therapists may be accessible. This will continue to be a concern as new generations of aspiring therapists are having their lives documented and uploaded by parents and loved ones, creating what may become fodder for searches by clients in the years to come.

Clinicians may never know if clients have access to personal information about them (Kolmes, 2012). Client motivations for seeking information about clinicians range from harmless curiosity to criminal intentions like stalking (Zur & Donner, 2009). Obviously, the motivations behind searches have implications for the course of the therapeutic relationship. In addition, they may influence how each practitioner engages not only with a particular client, but with the digital world as well.

For many of us, our personal lives have a digital component. In fact, it may be increasingly impossible to "escape having an online identity" (Nicholson, 2011). We engage with friends and family members online just as our clients do. We have interests that extend beyond our professional role and may necessitate online participation. Much like providers in small communities, we must each juggle the intersections with our clients in a way that allows us to exist socially as well as professionally in the "global village" connected by the "town square."

ROAD MAP FOR THE DIGITAL LANDSCAPE

The following recommendations are based on the technological realities present at the time of this writing and are intended to provide some ways for clinicians to engage digitally and to maintain their desired divide between personal and professional domains. The suggestions provide some guidance for operating in the digital space with competency in regard to social media sites and to online presence. The intention is that the recommendations serve as a starting point for clinicians with the awareness that as technology changes, so too must our knowledge of what is available; which mandates that providers continue to stay current with relevant ethical, legal, professional, and personal dynamics.

One of the first steps that a provider can take toward gaining control of their personal information is to identify what information is already available. This can be done by simply doing a search of one's own name on a search engine like Google. It is recommended that providers search for their names regularly to ensure that they are not inadvertently sharing information that they do not want to be public. To that end, it may be helpful to search for one's name in various forms. For example, "Dr. Jim Smith," "Dr. James Smith," "James Smith, Ph.D.," "Jim Smith, Ph.D.," and "Jim Smith and Indianapolis" might all be appropriate search terms. In the case of a person who has had a legal name change, it would be helpful to search for previous names as well to ensure that all personal information has been located. For those who would like to streamline the process of monitoring the availability of their personal information, Google has a notification option called Google Alerts. Google Alerts allows users to save searches and choose how frequently they would like a search to be completed. Once set up, searches will run on a schedule and the user will be notified of the information that is available about them (Zur & Donner, 2009).

It should be noted that, in addition to searching for names, it is possible to search for an image by using Google Images. Using this feature, it is possible to determine whether personal information is accessible and searchable through the use of a particular image of a provider. Individuals who have used a picture for both personal and professional purposes may find that an image search reveals information that was not accessible through a search of name or credentials. Therefore, it is recommended that providers also conduct searches on easily accessible images of themselves, such as a website photo or LinkedIn profile picture, especially if there is a chance that the photo has been used for nonprofessional purposes such as on a dating profile or a personal Facebook page (Kolmes, 2012).

Setting Up Privacy Protections

After conducting a thorough search of any name or photo that might lead to an inadvertent revelation of information, it is important to ensure that future information will be protected. One way to do this is to familiarize oneself of the privacy options that are available on common social networking sites. Understanding the options and potential pitfalls of the most common social networking sites can allow practitioners to determine whether they can effectively moderate the risks of inadvertent disclosure to their own satisfaction.

Facebook—Personal Pages

Facebook, a common social and business networking site, is used by many people to connect and relate to individuals in their personal and social lives. In keeping up with common concerns that Facebook users expressed about privacy, Facebook has recently increased the control that users can have over their personal information (Facebook, 2015). In fact, Facebook users have a considerable number of tools to ensure that their privacy remains intact. However, the default settings when signing up for the service permit much more information to be viewed than most practitioners would knowingly allow.

Understanding the meaning of the options that are available can allow practitioners to select the amount of privacy that they desire. Facebook options allow users to decide who can see past and future posts that they make. It should be noted that leaving a profile completely public will allow any person to access all, or nearly all, of the pictures and posts that have existed on the profile since it was established. On the other hand, a practitioner who allows only their "friends" to see their posts should be aware that this does not guarantee that people connected to their friends (friends of friends) will not see the post. Friends of friends may also be able to view photos or comments in which a user is tagged, which is why it is important to be diligent about utilizing all of the available privacy options.

Lehavot, Barnett, and Powers (2010) wrote about the potential pitfalls of accepting "friend requests" from clients given the likelihood that such a connection could result in a potentially harmful multiple relationship. Additionally, accepting a friend request would also create a loss of privacy for both client and therapist. However, settings are available to strengthen privacy and reduce accidental loss of privacy for both the therapist and client. See Table 5.3 for recommendations regarding how users can configure their Facebook accounts to obtain an optimal level of privacy (Facebook Help Center, 2015).

In many cases, these settings will prevent practitioners from receiving friend requests from their clients. However, if a client happens to have a

Table 5.3 Facebook: Optimal Privacy Settings—Personal Users

Setting/feature	*Optimal privacy*	*Special considerations*
Future posts	"Only me" or "friends"	Allowing friends to see posts does add some possibility that friends of friends might gain access to some content.
Limit past posts	"Only me" or "friends"	
Who can send friend requests	"Friends of friends"	Reduces the chance that clients will be able to send you a friend request.
Who can send private messages	Basic OR strict filtering	Strict filtering allows you to specifically choose who can send you messages while basic filtering will generally allow only your friends to send you private messages.
Who can search you by email/ phone #	"Friends"	Prevents clients from using contact information to locate your Facebook profile.
Can search engines link to your timeline	No	Prevents Facebook content from appearing when a person looks up your name on the Internet.
Who can post to your timeline	"Only me" or "friends"	Prevents unwanted posts.
Review post/picture before added to timeline	On	Allows user to have control of content that is posted about them.
Who can follow you	"Friends"	Prevents clients from accessing your personal information.
Who sees tag suggestions on pictures that look like you	"No one"	Prevents your name from being suggested for others to tag you.
Friend requests	Accept requests from people you know personally	Protects your personal information from being seen by current and prospective clients.

connection in common with the practitioner, they may still be able to send a friend request to their provider. If a practitioner knows that a client has a personal connection in common with them, they have the option to "Block" that user. Blocking a user will prevent both the client and practitioner from seeing content that is generated by the other and will also disallow "Friend requests" and private messages. This is the most secure way to protect private information from a particular individual if it is known that an overlap exists. However, practitioners may not be aware of a shared connection. Therefore, it is recommended that providers approach this matter by monitoring and maintaining their own privacy as well as by initiating policies that clearly indicate how they will approach such situations when they occur. Since clients may not understand the impact of connecting on social media, therapists should discuss their decision to decline/block a connection with a client.

Facebook—Business Pages

Facebook users also have the option of creating a business page, which can be used to help clinicians post mental health-related material, promote a specialty, and develop their own personal brand. Facebook business pages function quite differently from personal Facebook pages. One of the primary differences between a personal and a business page is that businesses do not have "friends." Instead, page visitors have the option of "liking" the page. When users like the page, they will receive updates as the business posts information (Facebook Help Center, 2015). Currently, there is no way to prevent clients from liking a business page, which may leave practitioners confused about the ethical responsibilities that this activity might require. Kolmes (2009) indicated that unlike "friend" connections, a "like" does not constitute a two-sided relationship and clients are free to disclose their own connection to providers even though providers are required to maintain a client's confidentiality. Providers do have a responsibility to ensure that clients have a clear understanding of the potential impact of making a public connection or posting a review about their services but, inevitably, it is the client's choice. Clients should also be made aware that it is possible to privately receive updates regarding the activity of a business page without "liking" the page. This can be achieved by subscribing to the Short Message Service (SMS) or Rich Site Service (RSS) updates (Kolmes, 2009).

A challenge on Facebook business pages involves clients posting messages. Clients are able to post some comments and reviews without restrictions. This allows for the possibility that clients may identify themselves as clients or make suicidal or homicidal statements. However, steps can be taken to reduce the risk of this happening. Suggestions are listed in Table 5.4 for ways to obtain a maximum amount of security and to prevent most messages from being visible to the public on the page (Facebook Help, 2015). It should be noted that even if messages are hidden from the page, they will still be seen by the provider who may have a duty to act if such messages include suicidal or homicidal content.

Overall, Facebook has many safeguards that allow users to protect their personal information. When used to their full potential, they can provide

Table 5.4 Facebook: Optimal Privacy Settings—Business Page Users

Option/feature	*Optimal privacy*	*Special considerations*
Visitor posts	"Disable posts by other people on the page."	This does not prevent all messages.
Messages	"People cannot contact my page privately."	To prevent clients from sending you private messages.
Tagging ability	"Only people who manage my page can tag photos on it."	To prevent posting of pictures by personal connections.
Page moderation (for risk management)	"Posts containing these words are blocked."	Consider adding words such as: suicide, kill, kill myself, dead, death, cut, cutting, abuse, live etc.
Page moderation (to block most comments)	"Posts containing these words are blocked."	Consider adding words such as: a, and I, we, them, they, he, she, are, what, who, then, why, the, LOL, etc.
Banned users—clients	Any known clients who might post problematic content OR all clients who might post comments.	Note: If those clients try to post, they will be sent a message indicating that they are not permitted to comment.
Banned users—personal connections	Any person who you want to separate from potential exposure to the public or your clients.	Consider adding parents/children/loved ones. Their pages may be more public and may reveal information about you.

users with reasonable protections against unwanted disclosures of information. Users should be aware that as the privacy options change from year to year, previous privacy settings may be impacted. Therefore, settings should be reviewed regularly so that protections remain strong to ensure that unwanted information is not publicly available.

LinkedIn

LinkedIn, a popular professional networking site, allows users to make professional connections, post resumes, and keep in contact with individuals in their professional circles. LinkedIn allows users to express and display their professional goals and may be a place where professionals attempt to develop and reinforce their own professional brand. However, another common aspect of LinkedIn is that it actively approaches a user's connections for endorsements. This may leave some practitioners wondering how they can promote a business presence without violating ethical standards that mandate that psychologists not solicit testimonials from clients (American Psychological Association, 2010). However, LinkedIn has made it possible to disable endorsements, making it possible to promote oneself without fear that a client will feel obligated to provide an endorsement of a provider's skills. Table 5.5 contains suggestions for optimizing privacy (LinkedIn Help Center, 2015).

Table 5.5 LinkedIn: Optimal Privacy Settings

Option/feature	*Optimal privacy*	*Special considerations*
Who can see your connections	"Only you."	Your 1st degree connections can always see your connections.
Connection requests	Add people that you know personally or professionally.	Avoids access to your information by current or prospective clients.
Who can follow your updates	"Your connections" OR "everyone."	Depends upon your use of LinkedIn (primarily personal or professional use).
Blocking	Block all individuals whose connection is problematic.	Some of your public information is still available to blocked users.
Who can search you by using your phone number	"1st degree connections."	Helps prevents clients from locating your profile using your phone number.
Data sharing with third party applications	Off	Prevents applications from using your contacts and connections for advertising purposes.
Endorsements	Off	Prevents LinkedIn from soliciting endorsements which may constitute a breach of ethical regulations.
Resume/vitae	Do not include personal phone number or address.	Resumés often include personal information such as a personal cell phone number or home address.
Summary	Avoid adding your personal phone number, address, or email address.	Information put in this section remains public regardless of other privacy settings.

Twitter

Twitter, a social networking site, allows users to post short updates about their thoughts, activities, and opinions. Twitter allows users to send instant messages and has been used by some professions as a mechanism for promotion. As with the other social media sites, it is important to understand how providers can use these services without compromising their professional lives by accidentally revealing personal information. To this end, Twitter has a number of mechanisms for creating a more private space. However, if you are found by a client, you will have difficulty screening your information since you can block users if they post inappropriate or harassing content on your profile. If practitioners choose to use Twitter personally, their best defense is to make every attempt to keep themselves from being found and identified by clients. Table 5.6 contains information on the features that are currently available to promote privacy (Twitter Help Center, 2015).

Table 5.6 Twitter: Optimal Privacy Settings

Option/feature	*Optimal privacy*	*Special considerations*
Location and bio	Leave blank.	Add only information that you wish to be publicly available.
Website address	Leave blank.	Add only if you want your professional identity to be connected to your Twitter presence.
Photo tagging	"Do not allow anyone to tag me in photos."	To prevent posting of pictures by personal connections.
Tweet privacy	"Protect my Tweets."	Allows control of who sees tweets. Past Tweets may continue to be visible.
Location	Do not check, "add location to my Tweets."	Consider also selecting, "delete all location information" to erase location from past tweets.
Searchability	Do not check, "Let others find me by my email address."	An email address, which might be easily accessed, can be used to find your personal information.
Blocking users	In order to block a person from posting inappropriate content, you can "block and report."	This feature cannot be used to keep a client from seeing your content. It can only be used to prevent a person from harassing you or posting inappropriately.

CONCLUSION

The speed at which change happens on the digital landscape occurs so quickly that it is leaving many of us scrambling to keep up. Private practices and individual providers are left trying to operate in an environment that is anything but static. The authors of this chapter acknowledge that even as this book goes to press, many new challenges will be emerging as the technology changes. As those challenges develop, practitioners will find that navigating changes will require pursuance of education about the technology while holding onto the basic core ethical and legal tenets of our profession. Rooted in a solid ethical and legal foundation, providers can be informed and proficient participants in the digital landscape.

REFERENCES

American Counseling Association. (2014). American Counseling Association Code of Ethics. Retrieved on 7/11/2015 from http://www.counseling.org/resources/aca-code-of-ethics.pdf.

American Psychological Association. (2013). Guidelines for the practice of telepsychology. *American Psychologist, 68*(9), 791–800. doi: http://dx.doi.org/10.1037/a0035001.

American Psychological Association. (2010). Ethical principles of psychologists and code of conduct. Retrieved from http://www.apa.org/ethics/code/principles.pdf.

Anderson, S.C. & Guyton, M.R. (2013). Ethics in an age of information seekers: A survey of licensed healthcare providers about online social networking. *Journal of Technology in Human Services, 31*(2), 112–128. doi: 10.1080/15228835.2013.775901.

Baker, D.C. & Bufka, L.F. (2011). Preparing for the telehealth world: Navigating legal, regulatory, reimbursement, and ethical issues in an electronic age. *Professional Psychology: Research and Practice, 42*(6), 405–411. doi: http://dx.doi.org/10.1037/a0025037.

Bradley, L.J., Hendricks, B., Lock, R., Whiting, P.P., & Parr, G. (2011). Email communication: Issues for mental health counselors. *Journal of Mental Health Counseling, 33*(1), 67–79.

Clark, J. (2010). Social media and privacy. *Air Medical Journal. 29*(3), 104–107. http://dx.doi.org/10.1016/j.amj.2010.02.005.

Facebook. (2015). Company info: Stats. Retrieved on 7/11/2015 from https://newsroom.fb.com/company-info/.

Facebook Help Center. (2015). Basic privacy settings and tools. Retrieved on 07/11/2015 from https://www.facebook.com/help/privacy/basic-controls.

Harris, S.E., & Robinson Kurpius, S.E. (2014). Social networking and professional ethics: Client searches, informed consent, and disclosure. *Professional Psychology: Research and Practice, 45*(1), 11–19. doi: http://dx.doi.org/10.1037/a0033478.

Health Insurance Portability and Accountability Act of 1996, 42 U.S.C. § 1320d-9 (2010).

Kolmes, K. (2009). Managing Facebook as a mental health professional. Retrieved on 7/11/2015 from http://drkkolmes.com/2009/06/08/managing-facebook-as-a-mental-health-professional/.

Kolmes, K. (2012). Social media in the future of professional psychology. *Professional Psychology: Research and Practice, 43*(6), 606–612. doi: http://dx.doi.org/10.1037/a0028678.

Kolmes, K. & Taube, D.O. (2014). Seeking and finding our clients on the Internet: Boundary considerations in cyberspace. *Professional Psychology: Research and Practice, 45*(1), 3–10. doi: http://dx.doi.org/10.1037/a0029958.

Lehavot, K., Barnett, J.E., & Powers, D. (2010). Psychotherapy, professional relationships, and ethical considerations in the myspace generation. *Professional Psychology: Research and Practice, 41*(2), 160–166. doi: http://dx.doi.org/10.1037/a0018709.

LinkedIn. (2015). Newsroom: about us. Retrieved on 7/11/2015 from https://press.linkedin.com/about-linkedin.

Linked In Help Center (2015). Account security and privacy: Best practices. Retrieved on 7/11/2015 from https://help.linkedin.com/app/answers/detail/a_id/267.

Nicholson, I.R. (2011). New technology, old issues: Demonstrating the relevance of the Canadian Code of Ethics for Psychologists to the ever-sharper cutting edge of technology. *Canadian Psychology, 52*(3), 215–224. doi:10.1037/a0024548.

Perrin, A. & Duggan, M. (2015). Americans' Internet access: 2000–2015. Pew Research Center. Retrieved from http://www.pewInternet.org/files/2015/06/2015-06-26_Internet-usage-across-demographics-discover_FINAL.pdf.

Poeppelman, T. & Blacksmith, N. (2014). Personal branding via social media: Increasing SIOP visibility one member at a time. *TIP: The Industrial-Organizational Psychologist, 51*(3), 112–119.

Privacy Settings and Safety Tips for Socializing on Twitter. (2015). Retrieved on 07/11/2015 from http://www.fightcyberstalking.org/privacy-settings-twitter/.

Twitter. (2015). Twitter usage/company facts. Retrieved on 7/11/2015 from https://about.twitter.com/company.

Twitter Help Center. (2015). Help center. Retrieved on 7/11/2015 from https://support.twitter.com.

Zur, O. & Donner, M.B. (2009). The Google factor: Therapists' transparency in the era of Google and MySpace. *The California Psychologist.* Retrieved on 7/11/2015 from http://www.zurinstitute.com/search.html?q=google%20factor.

Zur, O. (2014). Record-keeping of phone messages, email and texts in psychotherapy & counseling, online publication, Zur Institute. Retrieved on 7/09/2015 from http://www.zurinstitute.com/digital_records.html.

Chapter 6

Integration of Clinical Healthcare Strategies

Preparing Clinicians for Shifting Roles

Kristy M. Fritz-Bosse and Jennifer M. Ossege

The need for integration of healthcare services continues to grow, and behavioral health practitioners must be aware of the ways in which treatment can be more effective when utilizing an interprofessional approach. As the need for health psychology services develops, there are opportunities for practitioners to expand their knowledge base into new methods of service delivery. It is imperative that behavioral health providers are able to interact effectively with the medical community, and that they position themselves as reputable, competent colleagues with an integrated knowledge base. While not all professionals are able to provide fully integrated care, there are many levels of collaboration, including offering regular referral streams, providing consultations or urgent appointment availability, co-locating services, and even setting up a fully integrated practice. The focus of this chapter will be on providing guidance and strategies for the clinician in private practice to enhance collaboration and improve patient care. For example, it is important for clinicians to become familiar and comfortable with the medical culture's norms and expectations (e.g., brief and concise updates, and changing language from "client" to "patient" to better fit the biopsychosocial model), as well as the use of health and behavior codes, brief treatment approaches, and opportunities to provide health psychology consultations.

WHAT IS INTEGRATED CARE, AND HOW DOES IT APPLY TO ME?

Over the years, various models have been proposed that attempt to best explain the idea of integrated service delivery, but inconsistencies still exist. The concept of collaborative care may best be understood as a continuum (Blount, 2003; Blount, Shoenbaum, Kathol, Rollman, Thomas, O'Donohue, & Peek, 2007; Kessler & Stafford, 2008).

Table 6.1 Collaborative Care Continuum

Coordinated care model	*Co-located model*	*Integrated care model*
Primary care and behavioral health providers maintain separate facilities, delivery of care, billing, etc. Collaboration on patient cases occur on an as-needed basis. Good referral relationship.	Medical and behavioral health services are located in the same facility. Communication occurs regularly and some face-to-face collaboration occurs. Generally, separate records and treatment plans are maintained.	Behavioral health providers and primary care providers work alongside each other in care delivery. They work on the same treatment plan and generally share medical records.

On one end of the continuum exists a *coordinated care model*, consisting of primary care providers and behavioral health providers who maintain separate facilities, delivery of care, billing, etc., and collaborate on cases only on an as-needed basis. In this type of care, there is often a good referral relationship, and information is generally shared as situations arise that require collaboration between providers. A *co-located model* falls in the middle of the continuum, and generally is described as a system in which medical and behavioral health services are located in the same facility, with communication occurring regularly between the providers (often informally). There may be some face-to-face time spent in collaboration as well, but generally the providers maintain separate treatment plans and records. On the other end of the continuum exists the *integrated care model*, which truly is a fully integrated approach in which behavioral health providers are working alongside primary care physicians (and often other healthcare professionals) in a shared system, working with the same treatment plan, collaborating to deliver care, and generally using the same database or shared medical record (Hunter, Goodie, Oordt, & Dobmeyer, 2014; Oss, Braunstein, & Brock, 2015).

Clinicians in the private practice world may wonder why this is important. Why should we pay attention to this developing shift in the delivery of services? Many providers in the private practice sector have ignored this changing climate. While the need for mental health providers in more traditional settings likely will not go away anytime soon, it is important to understand what changes are occurring so that private practitioners can determine how best to respond and to prepare for the new culture of healthcare as it is growing in frequency of practice.

The Patient Protection and Affordable Care Act of 2010 has brought numerous provisions which mental health professionals should have a working knowledge of. It is important to understand the changing landscape of our healthcare system in order to truly understand the importance of integrated care, and why we must get on board as mental health practitioners in private practice. According to Suzanne Bennett Johnson, Ph.D., "Integrated care is the exact opposite of our current system: It is patient-centered care, and it rejects mind/body dualism" (Clay, 2012, p. 62). The healthcare reform law emphasizes a push toward patient-centered care, and calls for integration of behavioral health and primary care (Clay, 2012). However, there has not been any formalized standardization in terms of models of integration, and other variables, such as financial outcomes, are in need of continued monitoring.

Mental health clinicians, including psychologists, need to begin to identify as *healthcare providers,* and become full partners in the healthcare system (Bray, 1996; Frank, McDaniel, Bray, & Heldring, 2007). As Bray (2010) comments, "In some respects, we as a profession are in uncharted waters, often unable to see ahead because of the huge economic forces and policy changes at work" (p. 365). The political and economic climates will greatly influence this movement, and we have to be willing to embrace change as a profession. It is helpful to have some working knowledge of what is happening secondary to the healthcare reform, in order to more fully embrace the idea of change, and to understand the changes that are happening within the behavioral healthcare and medical fields.

Patient-centered medical homes (regular sources of care that are multifaceted and are based on a relationship between the patient and the physician) are becoming the expectation, which is a clear example of where integrated healthcare applies. The "medical home" is strongly supported in research, and the real purpose of a medical home is to help patients receive quality healthcare at a lower cost (Rosenthal, 2008), with better outcomes, and a higher level of patient satisfaction. Instead of patients receiving care in emergency rooms, walk-in clinics, or urgent care centers (which are often more costly and less effective), patients benefit from being managed in "medical homes" where there is a trusting partnership between patient, family, and provider (American Academy of Pediatrics, 2002).

Accountable Care Organizations (ACOs) are also gaining favor. ACOs are groups of healthcare organizations and professionals that come together to provide coordinated, high-quality care (Oss, Braunstein, & Brock, 2015). The general understanding is that healthcare provider organizations will be paid based on "value" of services provided. As clinicians, this is once again evidence that outcomes matter and will continue to drive reimbursement. Medical homes and ACOs have been used in the Medicaid and Medicare populations, and policies in these sectors often drive similar changes in the private sector. Therefore, it is important to understand the expectations that are emerging in terms of integrated care.

WHAT DOES THE ROLE OF THE INTEGRATED PSYCHOLOGIST LOOK LIKE?

The answer to this question greatly depends on the level of integration you want to establish. There are also several settings in which integrated care can occur: primary care, specialty medical clinics, long-term care settings, and community-based health settings. As mentioned above, there are various levels of integration that can exist. The role of the integrated behavioral healthcare provider may take various shapes depending on the model of integration, such as consultation/liaison, assessment, brief intervention, and program evaluation (American Psychological Association, 2015). There are many opportunities available for behavioral healthcare providers to get involved and engaged as part of the team of professionals providing services for the patients.

It is important to understand that nearly 70 percent of primary care visits are related to behavioral health needs (Fries, Koop, & Beadle, 1993). Primary care physicians have been dealing with behavioral health issues for some time, and this trend will only amplify. However, they often feel ill-equipped to do so, as their medical training has focused on treating issues that tend to be physiological in nature. Currently, even when the presenting problem is physiologically based, behavioral factors, such as stress, weight management, smoking, and alcohol consumption, frequently have a significant impact. Furthermore, shifts have been apparent in terms of psychotropic medications being prescribed primarily by primary care physicians. Often this is due to a shortage of available psychiatrists, as well as the tendency for the primary care physician to be the person whom the patient turns to for help. Again, many primary care physicians find themselves without an extensive knowledge base of psychotropic medications, and may feel as if they are out of their comfort zone treating psychiatric symptoms in isolation. For most medical providers, there is a great utility to having behavioral health providers with whom they can consult. Undeniably, there is a great need for behavioral healthcare professionals who understand integrated care and can effectively deliver services as such on an outpatient basis. In our experience, our physician colleagues have been more than eager to seek consultation on patient cases, and generally are very grateful for any amount of collaboration.

According to the American Psychological Association (2015), the role of the integrated psychologist may include conducting cognitive, personality, and behavioral health assessments, assisting in treatment of chronic medical conditions, diagnosing and treating mental and behavioral health issues, offering consultation and recommendations to healthcare providers and relatives of patients, developing team care strategies, measuring patient outcomes, and developing interventions.

Coordinated Care Model

As a private practitioner, the role of a consultant is a familiar one, but will look different than it might in a more fully integrated model where the behavioral health consultant might be readily available to the primary care physician. However, there are ways to promote collaboration between providers and to establish yourself as a trusted consultant even when operating from a coordinated care model. This may start simply by networking with area pediatricians and family medicine providers in order to create familiarity and credibility, as well as to establish referral relationships. While developing solid referral relationships is a lesser degree of integration than a behavioral health specialist working alongside a medical provider in primary care, it is still quite valuable, and needs to be a priority of all private practitioners. It is also important to communicate effectively and efficiently with the medical provider. In doing so, it is essential to consider your style of communication and ensure that it fits what the medical provider wants. The best way to make sure you are providing what they want is to ask about their communication preferences. Some will prefer quick telephone consults, while others find it helpful for you to provide updates in writing (which will likely become part of the patient's medical chart). In our experience, we have utilized communication forms that a large referring pediatric group developed and requested that we use as a means of consistent collaboration. Additionally, we find that taking the time to call and have a conversation with the medical providers is helpful in providing the best care. Sometimes, in coordinating care for a patient, a letter is not sufficient, and a phone conversation is necessary to effectively convey concerns. However, there are often challenges in achieving effective communications, such as coordinating phone calls during clinical care hours.

Some tips for communicating with medical professions include keeping your summaries concise and to the point, and clearly stating your questions and concerns. Medical professionals have very full patient loads and remain very busy. They often do not have time for a lengthy discussion about your theories about why the person is struggling with a specific issue. Keep it simple and to the point. Also, make it a priority to communicate with them. In the world of the medical professional, they send patients to specialists and they get a report back about the findings. Many do not have this same experience with mental health specialists, so this is your chance to stand out and do better. Not only is this practice likely to increase the satisfaction of both the physician and the patient, it will often turn into an increased stream of referrals to your practice.

In addition to working at developing good referral relationships with our outpatient, primary care colleagues, we have also found it beneficial to develop those relationships with inpatient behavioral health providers (often in the local pediatric hospital or nearby adult psychiatric units of area hospitals), as well as specialized outpatient medical clinics (e.g., adult renal transplant teams, pain clinics, etc.). In our experience, behavioral health specialists in inpatient settings are often looking for good referral sources that they can rely on in the community when patients are discharged home. Often, the behavioral health specialists working in the inpatient units are not able to follow all of the patients on an outpatient basis if or when follow-up services are needed. Having experience and training in working with patients with chronic health issues has been invaluable in terms of being able to market ourselves as a good fit for that specific need. Our experience has been that other providers will be more than eager to refer to us in private practice when we exhibit a collaborative spirit, willingness to work to have their patients seen in a timely manner, and demonstrate success in clinical outcomes. Communication is also important, particularly for ongoing medical concerns. Sometimes, it takes just one or two successful cases to keep you at the forefront in the minds of referral sources. Therefore, the time you spend delivering quality care and good communication will often be rewarded with increased referrals and a good community professional reputation.

Co-located and Integrated Care Models

In addition to the *coordinated care model,* there are growing opportunities for mental health professionals to implement *co-located* and *integrated care models,* particularly in primary care, and serving as consultants in this setting is likely the most practical approach for mental health providers to think about long-term. Those of us in private practice may find it useful to ease into the co-located or integrated care models. This may include renting office space in a medical setting, or perhaps working out an arrangement to see patients at the physician's office a few mornings a week.

Brief, concise assessments and interventions will be the norm in this setting. Although as mental health clinicians, we may be used to having 50- to 60-minute psychotherapy sessions with our clients and see them on a weekly or biweekly basis, in our role as a behavioral health specialist in a medical setting we have to be able to provide quick assessments and brief interventions. Many times our encounter with patients will be brief—as little as 15 to 30 minutes. We also have to be accessible to the physician. In our private practice world, our culture is to not interrupt a psychotherapy session, while in the medical arena, interruptions are frequent and should be expected. In order to be relevant to and appreciated by the primary care team, the mental health clinician has to be available. In addition to being readily available, any successful behavioral health consultant also has to be flexible and accommodating (Hunter, Goodie, Oordt, & Dobmeyer, 2014).

Often, in the initial phases of integrating services, mental health providers will need to spend time with their medical colleagues aimed at helping them understand their needs. What are the most common problems that they encounter in the primary care setting? Development of procedures and protocols may be a very important role of an integrated behavioral health clinician, particularly when trying to initially establish buy-in with our medical colleagues. Many times, they simply do not know what services we can offer. Letting them know how we can make their workload a bit lighter helps add value. They often do not have time to help someone through a panic attack, or to understand how to combat stress, or even to develop healthier eating habits. By letting the physicians know what you can offer to them and to their patients to enhance their care, you will establish your place on the team and demonstrate your value to them. Some behavioral health specialists will create handouts and other resources that serve the double role of informing the physician about their services while also helping the patient through a behavioral issue. Others may set up a lunch meeting with a brief presentation and discussion about what they may be able to offer in terms of assessment and services. Again, the focus, particularly at the beginning of your relationship with the medical professionals, is to show them how your services can help them provide better care and allow them to focus on the areas of medical practice that they enjoy most (Hint: Typically this is not the mental health side of practice!).

Other important tasks that the behavioral health provider can be involved in within an integrated setting include health promotion efforts, prevention of disease and injury, and management of chronic health issues. For example, in our private practice, we often work with children that a pediatrician has referred for ADHD assessment and brief intervention. As part of this interaction, we often focus on injury prevention when providing psychoeducation to parents. This may be something that the pediatrician does not always have time to do, but has been shown in research to be important in terms of injury prevention. Furthermore, we frequently work with patients with chronic health conditions and often spend considerable time coordinating care with their primary care physicians. Understanding and managing the psychological aspects of physical illness is critical to working more efficiently with the chronic illness population. It is important to understand the challenges that this population faces, such as difficulties with lifestyle change, adherence to medical regimens, cultural influences on health behaviors, and access to services. Specialized training in various health-related areas can be of great utility to the primary care physician who is looking for assistance with behavioral health matters.

As a consultant, or part of an integrated team, you will need to be familiar with the most common presenting issues in primary care, including anxiety, depression, sleep issues, and chronic diseases such as diabetes, obesity, and coronary heart disease. Mental health specialists are poised to offer services that are greatly needed for patients to make behavioral changes to enhance their health. Adherence is a major issue, and can contribute to substantial, negative health and financial outcomes when not appropriately addressed. Psychologists have specialized understanding of human behavior, motivation to change, and the effects of psychological factors on behavior, and yet often are not included on healthcare teams (Bray, 2010). There is undoubtedly a role for mental health professionals in the development and management of programs aimed at improving adherence.

Changes in Practice

The shift toward becoming an integrated care provider will likely make many practitioners very uncomfortable, as it can challenge the core approach to delivery of services that many have been using for years and have spent considerable time mastering. Let's face it, people often resist change, especially when the changes are unclear. Although some aspects of the delivery of care and the culture of practice are different within an integrated model, the skills and knowledge base that we have is easily transferred to this different setting.

Several of the key features of traditional mental health services, such as the luxury of a thorough assessment, in-depth case conceptualization, and even the idea of how the "clinical hour" looks, may be radically different at various levels of integration. Even the diagnostic process often feels rushed, as clinicians are expected to assess within a 15- to 30-minute time frame, rather than over an hour or even multiple 1-hour sessions, as may be typical in an outpatient mental health setting. This is perhaps one of the more challenging aspects to embrace, as we strive to be thorough and definitive in the diagnostic work-up. However, the pace in the medical world does not always allow for this, which can be rather unnerving to practitioners, and can create a sense of resistance. The changing landscape of mental health delivery, and of private practice in particular, demands that practitioners begin to migrate toward a new model, even if it puts us out of our comfort zone. Keep in mind that there will always be cases that require a more thorough diagnostic assessment than what can be competently completed in this setting and under this time pressure. As a consultant or behavioral health specialist, there will be times in which you will need to refer out to your colleagues in private practice or other settings to conduct a more thorough evaluation. These full psychological evaluations will still have a place, but they are not what is being asked of the integrated care specialist, who will rely more on screening and fast diagnostic skills.

From both our direct experience and our review of the literature, there are several key features of work within an integrated care model that will feel very different to the traditionally trained mental health clinician. Below are some key differences between traditional private practice and a practitioner who is working within an integrated model of care.

Interventions Move Quickly

In an integrated care model, one must be willing to adjust to a fast-paced style. It is very different from the traditional setting in outpatient therapy where clinicians often spend 45 to 60 minutes with every patient. The "clinical hour" is simply incompatible with an integrated care model. The fast-paced nature of primary care is both exhilarating and tiring. Simply adjusting to the pace is often the most challenging aspect of working in an integrated care setting. In order to be successful in an integrated care model, you will also need to be very flexible, as physicians will call on you for a variety of reasons. You may have to be willing to expand the focus of your practice, often practicing within a generalist model, especially in primary care/family medicine. The ability to think on your feet is critical in this setting. Many people come to enjoy this fast-paced setting. However, it is not for everyone. Before venturing into the world of integrated care, you should consider the culture of seeing many patients for shorter amounts of time, as well as not knowing in advance much about the patient you will be seeing, and determine whether this is something that appeals to you. Remember, the need for long-term, private practice clinicians is not likely to vanish completely.

Additionally, the type of intervention in an integrated care setting is different. You will need to offer brief, succinct recommendations (Hunter, Goodie, Oordt, & Dobmeyer, 2014). The assessment and intervention processes happen quickly, versus in a traditional outpatient mental health setting where several sessions may be used to get a "clinical feel" for what is going on. Adopting a solution-focused approach will be critical in working within an integrated care model. According to Hunter, Goodie, Oordt, and Dobmeyer (2014), there are several key interventions that are effective in addressing a host of presenting concerns common in primary care: relaxation training, goal setting, cognitive disputation, motivational interviewing strategies, problem solving, self-monitoring, behavioral self-analysis, stimulus control, and assertive communication. Many of these interventions are ones familiar to traditionally trained mental health providers. The method of delivery is simply different, in that the window of opportunity is much smaller. Hunter, Goodie, Oordt, and Dobmeyer (2014) propose that behavioral health clinicians need to be able to deliver effective interventions in one to four

30-minute appointments. While many traditional mental health providers are becoming more accustomed to brief psychological interventions and time-limited treatment, the aforementioned parameters can feel overwhelming. However, many find that with practice and a sharpening of their skills, they are able to work effective treatment into this window of time. It can be helpful to have many resources on hand so that you can provide the patient with specific skills, information, strategies, or techniques to help them be most effective in following up with your recommendations.

Keep It Brief

As mental health professionals, we are often criticized for the manner in which we speak and the language that we use. It is not uncommon to hear complaints that we use too much psychological jargon or "psychobabble." Be concise and allow brevity to be your friend. For many of us, this is challenging, as we have traditionally been trained to write thorough and detailed assessment reports. After all, in our graduate training, we were often reinforced for lengthy descriptions and thorough assessments. However, in the changing landscape of psychological practice, we have to learn to adopt a medical style of presenting cases, giving feedback, and providing documentation. Remember to be brief and to the point. You have to learn to be succinct to survive in the medical world. It is also important to pay attention to wording. For example, small but meaningful changes, such as referring to "patients" versus "clients," can be very important in more fully integrating into the culture. Calling their patient your client can be confusing to them, and implies that you are not working on the same team. Using a shared term (such as "patient") helps to close the gap. Integrated care providers have to be flexible and willing to make these simple but important adjustments in order to successfully collaborate with the medical world.

Know the Medical Lingo

Additionally, knowing the lingo within the medical culture will assist you in communicating more effectively with other care providers, as well as with patients. Familiarity with medical terminology, procedures, etc., can go a long way in establishing your credibility with medical practitioners. It may be helpful to begin familiarizing yourself with medical terms and procedures by subscribing to a medical journal or newsletters. This can help increase your knowledge base and help you get to know the lingo. However, it is also important that you do not force this or overstep your professional role or boundary. This can be very off-putting to our medical colleagues, and can also bring up ethical questions.

Be Realistic

It is imperative that, as a behavioral health clinician, you set realistic expectations for your acceptance into the medical world. Know that some physicians are much more open-minded about integration than others, even within the same practice setting. Thankfully, we think it is fair to say that openness to behavioral health, and working alongside our medical colleagues, is becoming much more of the trend, and most medical teams will welcome you with open arms. However, expect that you may face some resistance, and try not to be too defensive about it. It may be helpful to know that in the medical setting there is typically a hierarchy, and do not be surprised to learn that mental health professionals are not at the top. Many medical professionals will become more accepting of the role of behavioral health specialists as they see the benefit for their patients and themselves.

Make Yourself Added Value to the Practice

Proving your value is a concept that you must embrace when working in the medical system. This takes time and persistence. You may need to change the minds of some staff members, nurses, and even the physicians. However, it is our experience that if you prove your utility just once, they will come back! You may feel at times like you are shamelessly promoting your worth as a practitioner. Do not force it, but understand that, in general, most people do not truly understand what a good mental health professional can bring to the table, particularly within the medical setting. Try like hell to be successful, which will get their attention and lead to future referrals/consultation requests. Be personable, develop a thick skin, and do not get offended when you think your services have not been valued. Working within the medical model can be challenging. Mental health is still misunderstood and undervalued, but fortunately residency programs are requiring training in behavioral health, and foster more psychological mindedness as part of physician training. Many newer physicians are accustomed to mental health professionals working side-by-side with them. It has also been our experience that often medical providers that have been in the industry longer have come to really value us simply due to the fact that psychological issues are such a part of presenting problems seen in primary care. Since patients often struggle to find psychotherapists and psychiatrists that accept their insurance and/or are taking new patients, they often rely on their primary care provider to help them deal with their psychological issues.

Despite these great advances, be realistic, and remember that you may be another "step" or hassle for some staff (i.e., nursing staff/PCAs), who may not value or understand your role. It can feel like a hassle to them to have to explain your involvement to patients, especially if they don't understand your purpose. Try to gain an understanding of the culture within the office, tread lightly, and be aware of "turf wars." In our past experiences in inpatient medical settings and primary care, we have often been called upon to work with patients during medical procedures (e.g., pain management, distraction, etc.). You will face complacency and staff who do not welcome change. Your presence in the clinic/office may be a threat to staff or a drain on resources. They may take your intervention as a commentary that they aren't interacting with the patients effectively enough, and now behavioral health has been consulted to improve procedures. Work to gain allies, and in time they will appreciate your worth. Find those who are championing your cause and are supportive of your interventions, and also be aware of the decision makers who may attempt to block your successes.

ADVANTAGES OF INTEGRATED CARE

There are several advantages to the integration of physical health and mental healthcare. Notably, expenditures take a front seat. There is clear evidence that insurance companies will save money when an integrated system is in place (Chiles, Lambert, & Hatch, 1999; Olfson, Sing, & Slesinger, 1999). It has been well-documented that integrated care models result in less emergency room visits, reduced length of stay when hospitalized, and less medication use for patients (Oss, Braunstein, & Brock, 2015).

As part of the Patient Protection and Affordable Care Act, there is now a substantial amount of provisions in effect that will drive healthcare delivery. For example, Medicaid health homes and Accountable Care Organizations in Medicare are standard. Pay-for-performance models are emerging, and providers will be penalized for patients with high rates of hospital readmissions (Oss, Braunstein, & Brock, 2015). Additionally, it is likely that over the long term, providers will receive bonuses for achieving certain outcomes, particularly under payment models that focus on total cost of care or payment for value (Oss, Braunstein, & Brock, 2015). This should lead one to ask a couple of interesting questions. What are primary care providers going to need to do in order to obtain bonuses, and how might we, as psychotherapists, assist them in that goal? What is my share going to be for helping achieve that goal? Will behavioral health specialists be evaluated in the same manner? How do I demonstrate my effectiveness as a clinician? Using outcome measures, including patient satisfaction measures, is an important step in collecting data to support the efficacy of treatment.

One the most critical factors to consider in the changing landscape of healthcare is, of course, cost. There is growing evidence that coordinated care lowers overall healthcare expenditures. The bottom line is, this matters and is going to be a driving force over time. In addition to lowering overall costs, integrated care improves patient access to services and contributes to improved quality of care, as well as increased patient satisfaction. There is improved ease of communication between providers and better continuity of care for patients.

Ultimately, integrated care is emerging as what helps patients, what payor sources are looking to fund, and what physicians are going to expect. As private practice providers, we have got to find a way to fit into this model. It is imperative that we embrace the change from mental health professionals to healthcare professionals, and are open to receiving specialized training on how to work closely with primary care physicians (Frank, McDaniel, Bray, & Heldring, 2007). It is still somewhat of a niche market that demands well-trained clinicians that understand the unique challenges of this population. Ultimately, healthcare is moving to a value-based system, and it is imperative that psychotherapists deliver excellent care and are able to show good outcomes in order to survive the changing climate.

Without a doubt, another major advantage of integrated care is also the ease of "handing off" patients. Many physicians don't want to have to manage mental health, but they are being forced to do so by the shifts within healthcare. Many physicians appreciate the immediacy of on-the-spot consultation with a behavioral health specialist, or at least appreciate a streamlined referral process. Furthermore, patients generally respond well to the live "hand-off." Often, it facilitates patient follow-up if they can meet the provider, and patients often report that they are more open to meeting with a behavioral health specialist in the "space" they already know. In fact, many behavioral health specialists provide services within a traditional exam room, as it is familiar territory for the patient, and eases the portability of the therapist to go where needed. While it can take some getting used to, many clinicians enjoy the simplicity that this offers. Further, our experience has also been that patients report less stigma about receiving behavioral health intervention when this is part of their medical care, and/or when their physician has recommended the provider. After all, instead of being referred to "mental health" or to a "psychotherapist," they are referred to a "behavioral health specialist." Language can make a difference when it comes to breaking down stigma and resistance to treatment. In addition, many patients are more open to treatment following a warm hand-off and introduction from their physician. Credibility is typically automatically established, and it generally doesn't feel like "starting from scratch" with someone new. This often allows the behavioral health specialist to move quickly to the intervention and make the most of the time provided. When speaking specifically about behavioral health services within primary care, whether simply a co-location or truly integrated model, patients tend to like the "one-stop shopping" experience.

COMMON PRESENTING PROBLEMS

As a psychotherapist working across the three proposed models of integrated service delivery, you will witness various presenting issues. Behavioral health specialists will be consulted to assist physicians in dealing with the most common behavioral health problems, such as depression and anxiety (Bray, 1996). For psychotherapists working in a more fully integrated model, many patient issues will be related to adherence to medical regimens, coping with disease management, and overall adjustment to the medical issue (adjustment to the disease process, medical regimen, daily activities, and school/work performance). Further, managing chronic pain is a common patient scenario, and this often contributes to physicians referring to mental health, whether in-house or out in the community. Behavioral health professionals are also frequently consulted when there is recognition that a psychological disorder presents as a general medical condition. We find that this is a very common situation, particularly in pediatrics, and our medical colleagues often refer children with chronic headaches, stomachaches, and other somatic issues when there is no appreciable, underlying medical etiology. One less common, but very important aspect to pay attention to when it presents itself, is medically related trauma and anxiety. This could be trauma experienced by a patient and/or family members. It could be related to things such as actual medical/procedural trauma, injury, anxiety about medical procedures, or even trauma related to receiving healthcare information and/or an initial diagnosis. Lastly, across all models of integrated service delivery, mental health professionals need to address family systems, school (specifically school reentry), peers, employers, and the unique dynamics involved for patients with chronic health concerns, as well as patients' relationships with their families and caregivers.

MANAGING UNIQUE CHALLENGES IN PRIVATE PRACTICE

As a practitioner who works within any one of these proposed service delivery models, it is possible that you will have more clinical contact with patients with chronic illness. This means that they are prone to flare-ups with pain or illness more often than other patients you may see in a traditional mental health setting. While this may not immediately seem to be a big deal, you must consider how to be fair about missed appointments when working with these patients. Often, they have more barriers in terms of adherence to treatment, including showing up for appointments. Another issue is that they often have numerous medical visits, which may require you to be somewhat flexible in terms of appointment times in order to help the patient reduce the amount of missed school or work.

In moving toward integrated care, psychotherapists may also find that they are faced with unique situations that can possibly lead to ethical dilemmas and/or legal issues (e.g., bioethics, genetic testing). While we are accustomed to dealing with ethical dilemmas in the practice of mental health, we must stay mindful about such possibilities in the medical world, even if our physician colleagues do not necessarily view ethical situations through the same lens.

Engaging in outreach and collaboration takes time, and building relationships is not always easy work, but keep in mind that this is part of our skill set as mental health professionals. For the clinician in private practice, the reality is that time spent in collaborative efforts, specialized training, etc., means less time in the office seeing patients and generating revenue. However, it is critical that we put in the effort to build collaborative relationships. As you work to sell the value of your services, you may find that you have to be willing to devote a significant amount of unpaid time to securing your place as a behavioral health specialist. One example of this may be educating your physician colleagues on screening tools that they could incorporate in clinical practice with patients. Primary care physicians often report increased satisfaction in the management of particular behavioral health issues, such as Attention-Deficit/Hyperactivity Disorder (ADHD), when screening tools are available (Tynan, 2015). However, the long-term benefit in establishing credibility, buy-in for services, and the appreciation of the value that you bring to the practice, as well as increased referrals, can often make this initial expenditure of time worthwhile in the long run.

WORKING OUT THE KINKS

There are several complicating factors that will need to be worked out as psychotherapists move toward more fully integrated care. For example, record sharing is just one issue that needs to be addressed. There are often concerns from psychotherapists working in medical communities about the confidentiality of information recorded in the medical chart. There are various approaches to dealing with this, but certainly it is an issue that will need to be addressed as you consider integrated care. On a legal front, who owns the record? Are there measures taken to protect confidential psychological information, substance abuse information, etc., particularly if records are released? Who has access to the records? Who has access to release records? If interface is allowed, how are mental health data going to be protected? All of these are questions that (at the time of this writing) have yet to be fully answered.

Billing and payment is perhaps one of the more complicated issues when one thinks of working in an integrated fashion and, again, this will vary greatly depending on the service delivery model that one is using. Many behavioral health practitioners still report that they face challenges in receiving consistent reimbursement from Health and Behavior (H&B) billing codes. It is concerning that while the H&B codes are often the most appropriate billing codes to use, many practitioners are still receiving denials of coverage, and appeals, even those that include evidence of cost-saving benefits of services captured with H&B codes, often do not yield reversals of insurance denials (Duke, Guion, Freeman, Wilson, & Harris, 2012). The reality simply remains that insurance authorizations and payment are barriers that will require on-going focus and advocacy.

SUMMARY

While the professional ground continues to shift beneath our feet, there are opportunities for individuals currently in private practice to get involved in and become a part of the movement toward integrated care. There is no need to fear the loss of private practice, as it appears there will always be a place for it in the future. However, it is important and appropriate to pay attention to what is happening all around us, and to prepare ourselves for changes in the delivery of mental health or behavioral health services. There are some challenges yet to be overcome, largely in terms of logistics, but there is an exciting shift that can improve the outcomes, reduce the costs, and increase the satisfaction for patients.

Our goal in this chapter was to inform you of some of the ways in which services are being delivered in medical settings, and to describe some of the cultural differences between traditional private practice and what you can expect as you enter the world of integrated care. We also wanted to encourage you to learn more about integrated care, as this chapter only touches the tip of the iceberg of this large service delivery shift, and the available information is expanding every day. There is a growing amount of literature, workshops, trainings, online communities, etc., that all have the shared vision of integration of healthcare services. It is imperative that mental health providers understand these changes, prepare themselves for the changes, and embrace the opportunities that lie ahead.

REFERENCES

American Academy of Pediatrics. (2002). Policy statement: Organizational principles to guide and define the child health care system and/or improve the health of all children. *Pediatrics, 110*(1), 184–186.

American Psychological Association. (2015, June 22). Integrated health care. Retrieved from http://www.apa.org/health/integrated-health-care.aspx.

American Psychological Association. (2015, June 22). Health care reform: Integrated health care. Retrieved from http://www.apa.org/about/gr/issues/health-care/integrated.aspx.

Blount, A. (2003). Integrated primary care: Organizing the evidence. *Families, Systems & Health, 21,* 121–133.

Blount, A., Shoenbaum, M., Kathol, R., Rollman, B., Thomas, M., O'Donohue, W., & Peek, C. (2007). The economics of behavioral health services in medical settings: A summary of the evidence. *Professional Psychology: Research and Practice, 38,* 290–297.

Bray, J.H. (1996). Psychologists as primary care practitioners. In R.J. Resnick & R.H. Rozensky (Eds.). *To your health: Psychology across the lifespan* (pp. 89–100). Washington, D.C.: American Psychological Association.

Bray, J. (2010). The future of psychology practice and science. *American Psychologist, 65*(5), 355–369.

Chiles, J.A., Lambert, M.J., & Hatch, A.L. (1999). The impact of psychological interventions on medical cost offset: A meta-analytic review. *Clinical Psychology: Science and Practice, 6,* 204–220.

Clay, R. (2012). Integrated care is the future: Psychologists must make the case for working side by side with physicians. *Monitor, 43*(5), 62.

Duke, D., Guion, K., Freeman, K., Wilson, A., & Harris, M. (2012). Commentary: Health & behavior codes: Great idea, questionable outcome. *Journal of Pediatric Psychology, 37*(5), 491–495.

Frank, R., McDaniel, S., Bray, J., & Heldring, M. (2007). *Primary care psychology.* Washington, D.C.: American Psychological Association.

Fries, J., Koop, C., & Beadle, C. (1993). Reducing health care costs by reducing the need and demand for medical services. *The New England Journal of Medicine, 329,* 321–325.

Hunter, C., Goodie, J., Oordt, M., & Dobmeyer, A. (2014). *Integrated behavioral health in primary care: Step-by-step guidance for assessment and intervention.* Washington, D.C.: American Psychological Association.

Kessler, R. & Stafford, D. (2008). Introduction. In R. Kessler & D. Stafford (Eds.). *Collaborative medicine case studies: Evidence in practice* (pp. 3–8). New York, NY: Springer.

Olfson, M., Sing, M., & Slesinger, H.J. (1999). Mental health/medical cost care offsets: Opportunities for managed care. *Health Affairs, 18,* 79–93.

Oss, M., Braunstein, G., & Brock, I. (2015, April 7). Integrated care coordination and integrated service delivery models: Policy, regulation, financing, & practice in health & human services [Webinar]. In OPEN MINDS/Optum Webinar Series. Retrieved from https://www.openminds.com/.

Rosenthal, T. (2008). The medical home: Growing evidence to support a new approach to primary care. *Journal of the American Board of Family Medicine, 21*(5), 427–440.

Tynan, W. (2015, March 25). Increasing value through pediatric integrated care [Webinar]. In Kentucky Psychological Association Webinar Series: Integrating psychology and primary health care: Psychologists and physicians as collaborators. Retrieved from http://www.kpa.org/event/id/576319/Interactive-Webinar—Integrative-Care-Increasing-Value-Through-Pediat.htm.

PART II

CARING FOR THE CAREGIVER

Nourishing Yourself

Chapter 7

Isolation, Disconnection, and Burnout

The Importance of Staying Connected in Private Practice

Joy McGhee

THE BEAUTY OF PRIVATE PRACTICE

Embarking on the road towards private practice is a journey about which you have likely given much thought and consideration. Your ideas, questions, and concerns have taken up residence inside your head and may have at times been difficult to sort through. Even if your "elevator speech" does not yet completely answer the question, "Why do I want to be in private practice," it's likely that the following reasons have been a part of your thought process.

You Are the Boss

If you have ever heard a toddler fiercely assert their power by making the statement, "You're not the boss of me!" then you can probably appreciate how deeply rooted a personal sense of power is to many of us. The desire to be "in charge" of ourselves is natural and enhances our self-esteem and sense of self-efficacy. Most of us have had life experiences in which we have been subject to the ideas, moods, agendas, and whims of others, which sometimes leaves us wondering when our good ideas, stable moods, and creativity will have the opportunity to shine. Since much of our lives is spent in our professional work, having the opportunity to shape and mold that professional life becomes an integral aspect our experience.

The training required to become a mental health professional exposes us to a variety of service delivery settings, client populations, and colleagues. It is likely that you have encountered settings in which you felt immediately comfortable and established wonderful relationships with your colleagues and supervisors. During this type of experience there may have been alignment between your clinical/professional style and that of the facility. You may have felt that you were in the perfect place based on your needs and goals, and had complete confidence that your needs would be met and your goals realized. If you have experienced this professional bliss, count yourself among the lucky. An alternative to professional bliss (and something experienced by many of us) is the experience of being in a setting in which you encountered colleagues and supervisors who exemplified dysfunction and lacked the expected interpersonal competencies. Perhaps a pervasive and rigid theoretical orientation or organizational politics interfered with client care, and your attempts to improve an established system or look to the research to inform treatment approaches were met with resistance or misunderstanding. In fact, you may have had some supervisors from which you learned what not to do, rather than how to practice competently. If you have had this experience, you know how emotionally draining it can be and how it can cause us to question our choice of profession and wonder about the psychological health of our colleagues. In short, this might feel like a professional hell. It is probably easier to see why someone who had this experience would be more likely to run away screaming and vow to open their own practice so as to never be subject to such dysfunction again. While these descriptions obviously reflect the extremes of professional possibility, they are meant to demonstrate that very few experiences are completely perfect or hellish. No matter what your range of experiences have included, there have no doubt been times when you have been subjected to someone else's beliefs, ideas, and ways of understanding, and heard yourself say (probably in your head, but maybe out loud), "You're not the boss of me!" This may have been the beginning of your journey to private practice.

Making the decision to pursue private practice is significant and requires courage and conviction to move from, "You're not the boss of me" into, "I'm the boss of myself." Much of the first part of this book has focused on aspects of setting up a practice as well as the pros and cons of working in solo or group practices. However, within this chapter we will explore the reasons why it is essential to stay connected to various other professionals during your venture into the private practice world, as well as how to avoid feeling isolated, disconnected, and burned out.

If you have ventured out on your own into a solo practice, having the opportunity to be your own boss allows you to create something from scratch, or to refine something to your specifications. Being the boss means that you are the one who creates the framework for your professional life.

You decide what the guiding principles are, what your policies and procedures will be, and how you will brand yourself within your community. Being the boss means that when you have an idea, you can decide to put it into action, change direction if needed, and reap the benefits of its success. In addition to creating your own structure, being the boss also means that you have direct power over who else you invite into your practice. You can identify individuals who balance your weaknesses and complement your strengths, share your worldview, and communicate in ways that you understand. You are able to choose employees and/or business partners based on criteria that you deem important. These criteria could range from a shared love of Indian food to a visible commitment to issues of social justice within your community. The appeal of having control of and agency over your professional setting is undeniable and is often the initial prompt into private practice.

Some people enjoy the professional freedom that a private practice setting offers, but don't want to take on the business end of the daily operations of a practice. Many of these professionals find themselves better suited for joining a group practice, where they can generally still control their own schedules, client caseloads, and overall professional work, yet they share the expenses (and the burdens) of running a practice with other professionals or practice owners. Whether you are completely independent in your practice or you are a part of a group practice, many of the same principles apply.

Flexible Schedule

Many of us who are drawn to private practice have a strong desire and/or commitment to create and maintain a relatively healthy work-life balance. Frequently that means we are attempting to establish a successful professional life while still attending to partners, children, aging parents, or other outside interests, such as volunteer or advocacy work, or even hobbies. Additionally, some of us may be dealing with a personal chronic illness that requires our time and attention. During our training as clinicians, we had heard from many supervisors and workshop facilitators about the critical importance of self-care. Our professional activities can easily deplete our physical, mental, and emotional reservoirs, and without consistent engagement with the other parts of our lives, we can easily find ourselves depleted. Unfortunately, most corporate entities do not fully operate on this premise, and require us to work full-time schedules with little flexibility around our needs and desires to spend our time engaged with families and communities or attending to the management of chronic illness, having to carefully account for each hour away from work. Being in a private practice provides the freedom to create a schedule that can accommodate whatever external or internal demands we confront. Additionally, having a flexible schedule means that it can be adapted relatively easy when the demands of our lives change.

Outside of the personal benefits of a flexible schedule, many clients find it helpful to have the opportunity to receive services before or after their work schedules. Creating a private practice that acknowledges and meets the needs of a diverse clientele resonates with those practitioners who seek to serve diverse populations as well as those who understand the potential marketing benefits of offering nontraditional office hours.

Opportunity to Work with Specific Types of Clients

Every city is filled with clinicians who identify as "generalists," serving a wide range of clients and presenting problems. The role of the generalist practitioner is important, as they are willing and able to work with a variety of people, and make mental health services accessible to many individuals. After spending part of one's professional life working with the full range of presenting problems, you might find that there is a specific population or presenting problem with which you enjoy working. Developing a private practice allows you the opportunity to develop a niche or specialty in order to work with the types of issues and clients that you enjoy most. Your niche might be a specific disorder that you have focused on and developed a good deal of competence in, or it might be assessment-based, where you offer specific types of evaluations, or it could be working with a specific population that you have a great understanding about. You can develop your practice to be what you want it to be.

Income Potential

The issue of money, one of those subjects that we were always told was not discussed in polite company, continues to be a practical necessity and thus a significant point of consideration when anyone contemplates a professional endeavor. Conversations with colleagues will no doubt yield various perspectives about "income potential," but there still is money to be made in private practice. Figuring out how much money you want or need to make is obviously a personal decision and is impacted by many factors. In a private practice setting, you are in control of many of those factors. The aforementioned benefits of private practice, being the boss, flexible schedule, and the opportunity to work with specific types of clients are all contributing factors to the income potential of your private practice, as well as to your happiness in private practice.

THE DARK-SIDE OF THE UP-SIDE

Now that I have reminded you about the many factors that make private practice so great, it's important to consider the "dark-side of the up-side." This is not for the purpose of being a dark cloud over the beauty that can be private practice, but to expand your perspective, allowing you to see the full picture, not just the gilded frame surrounding it. This is especially important in considering how important it is to stay connected and to avoid the many pitfalls that are possible.

I'm the Boss = I Can't/Don't Want to Do It All

What about when you get what you want? You are the boss, which means you get the glory of independence and the agony of the responsibility. Not everyone is suited or prepared for what lies ahead when they decide to venture out on their own. As I stated earlier, it's not for everyone. Some people prefer the security of being in a group practice setting where the burdens are less. Consider Julia's experience:

> My plan, from the time I began graduate school, was to open a private practice and work with children and adolescents. I thought it would be relatively easy, especially since I was going to be the only decision maker. Once I found an office space, filled it with furniture, and began scheduling my first clients, I quickly realized that I had to deal with insurance companies for payment, I had to figure out how to get my name out into the community so I could attract more clients, I also had to find someone to do my billing and an accountant to handle my taxes...there was so much to do when I wasn't seeing clients, and it started to become overwhelming. This was new for me because I saw myself as a capable person, but there were so many decisions to make...I found myself wishing that I wasn't the boss.

I Have a Flexible Schedule = I'm Working Evenings and Weekends

Having a career that allows you to simultaneously stay connected and involved with your personal life is a wish come true for many people, and certainly a benefit of having your own practice and being in control of your own time. Operating outside of the demands of words like "productivity" and "client contact hours" brings a sense of relief and freedom. When you begin scheduling clients and other professional activities on days and times that are either convenient for you or the population of clients you're working with, it starts to become clear that the "convenient times" often occur in the evenings and weekends. This can be especially true when your clients are working adults, or children and adolescents who attend school during the day. There is nothing inherently wrong with working in the evenings or on the weekends, but when this schedule becomes the norm, it can result in missing out on the various family activities or personal care time that you intended to make available.

Opportunity to Work with Specific Types of Clients = Maybe I Shouldn't Be a Therapist

Let's face it, some days we may feel that we are the best therapist in the world, and other days it seems we are not effective as a therapist. There are ups and downs in private practice, just as there are in other clinical settings. It can lead to frustration, disappointment, and even burnout, particularly if we are going it alone in our professional worlds. Another therapist, Michael, shares his story:

> As I entered professional practice, I felt prepared to work with a variety of clients, but I had developed a special interest in working with couples. I would look at my schedule for the day and find myself looking forward to seeing the couples I had scheduled for that day. Over a period of a few months, I made the decision to focus on couples work and began accepting more of those referrals. Eventually I found myself with a practice that was 90 percent marital therapy, and the remaining 10 percent were adolescents and adults. For a little while I felt great satisfaction with the marital therapy I was doing, but of course I had some days where I thought very little was being accomplished. After a particularly difficult week, I found myself feeling very frustrated and ineffective, questioning my decision to work primarily with couples. When I tried to make sense of my deflated professional self-esteem, it occurred to me that without the variety of "less intense" and "more intense" clients, I was missing out on having a more balanced perspective; I was not getting enough of the positive, esteem-building experiences to balance out the difficult, deflating experiences.

Creating a professional niche has many advantages, and is often recommended during the course of graduate training. Identifying an area of expertise often brings a personal sense of competence and accomplishment. As you get known in the community for your specialty, it typically leads to increased referrals and the opportunity to provide consultation to colleagues who do not have your expertise. There are often requests for your specific skill set from potential clients. This can be a wonderful experience that leads to professional satisfaction and increased income potential; that is, until you begin to question your own competence and "calling" to be a helping professional. Spending too much time on any one thing can result in a myopic and distorted perspective of the "thing" and ourselves, and this fact is no different in private practice. All of us have "good days" where we have evidence of our positive impact on the lives of our clients. Sometimes this evidence comes from the client themselves in the form of a "Thank you," or, "I'm doing much better than I was when I first came to see you." Or even when we hear of word-of-mouth referrals from former clients, which is very gratifying. Other times the evidence is our own ability to be present with a grieving client, or helping a distressed parent better understand their angry, depressed teenager. Invariably, we also encounter the "difficult day," which is filled with poorly timed interventions and private thoughts of, "I have no idea what to say or do right now." The risk of working with the same client population or diagnosis day after day is encountering the same obstacles and challenges that are associated with that population and/or diagnosis. This increases the chances that we will question our training, our competence, our choices, even our clients, all of which eventually erode our energy.

What was initially a professional niche can sometimes morph into a professional ditch. Therefore, we have to consider the impact of finding a balance within our practice and work to not become isolated in our professional role.

Income Potential = I Don't Have Time or Knowledge to Market My Practice

Let's be honest, most (if not all) of us want our professional endeavors to be financially rewarding, but not many of us have received explicit directions on how to make that a reality. The initial start-up of a private practice is filled with the excitement of receiving new referrals and dedicating ourselves to providing excellent services to the consumers. If you have made the choice to accept private insurance, your client referrals likely come in a semiregular pattern, with predictable periods of high and low client contacts. During the slow periods, you may find yourself wondering how to attract more clients and/or how to get more referrals from the professionals in your local community. Thinking about it may be as far as you get, because the majority of your time and energy is being spent on other pressing matters, such as seeing clients, deciding how "flexible" your schedule will be for the next 2 weeks, trying to find the best price for Internet and phone service, negotiating better reimbursement rates with insurance carriers and asking the same insurance companies for authorization for more client sessions. Knowing how to successfully market your private practice takes intentional time and effort, for which you may not feel you have the time or expertise. Wanting or needing more clients, with little idea of how to accomplish that goal, simply adds more work to the "work" of private practice, and may contribute to experiencing financial concerns.

THE CALM BEFORE THE STORM

Have you ever told anyone, "Hindsight is 20/20?" This saying is frustrating, in part, because we know that everyone would avoid unpleasant consequences **IF** they were able to see them coming. If you could predict the "storms" that you would encounter as you planned to enter private practice, you would certainly prepare yourself with the appropriate gear.

Overwhelmed, Disillusioned, Uncertain, Unfulfilled

Whether you are "getting ready to get ready," or have already embarked upon opening your private practice, or have joined a group practice, hopefully there were parts of the preceding discussion that resonated with your experience or made you stop, think, and reflect on the thoughts and plans that you may have been considering. It's clear that private practice brings many professional and personal joys, but it can also bring feelings of isolation, professional loneliness, and disconnection from our colleagues. After all, we are bound by confidentiality and cannot talk about our clients to others in our personal lives. Even if we could, they are not likely to fully understand the work or the impact of the sessions on us as professionals.

The key to circumventing the rough road that can lead you to burnout is recognizing those initial feelings of isolation and paying attention to the impulse to talk to someone about that difficult session. Just like you took extra care to establish a firm structure for your practice—ideal location, accessible hours, reasonable and competitive fees, and contracts with insurance companies—it is imperative that you take extra care to establish a firm infrastructure as well. This infrastructure can be conceptualized as a framework that is established for the purpose of creating stability and providing protection for you, the most important aspect of your private practice.

Standing in the Rain with No Umbrella

Working in a private practice setting without a solid infrastructure of support is setting yourself up for some difficult times. Why should you have to know all of the answers? Whoever told you that you could do this all on your own (or that it would be a good idea to be on a professional island alone)? In many ways, going it alone in private practice is like standing in the rain without an umbrella. Recognize this as a choice—you can stand there getting wet and feeling miserable, or you can reach out and use an umbrella to protect you from the rain. I like to think about peer consultation as the umbrella that can protect us from isolation and burnout.

WHY IS PEER CONSULTATION IMPORTANT?

Intentionally integrating peer consultation into the infrastructure of a private practice provides the clinician with several advantages, all of which contribute to the well-being of both the clinician and the practice. When asked why they sought to be in a peer consultation group, Lewis, Greenburg, and Hatch (1988) found that clinicians reported reasons such as countering isolation and burnout, support for stress in private practice, learning therapeutic techniques, and exploring problematic attitudes towards clients. Discussion of ethical issues was also noted, and I would argue that it is our ethical responsibility as mental health professionals to engage in peer consultation so we can continue to develop and provide quality clinical care to our clients. Below, I will discuss many reasons why peer consultation should be an essential component to your private practice, including ethics, professional and social connection, networking, and other business opportunities.

Ethics

Every helping professional is subject to the ethics and code of conduct of their governing body. The Ethical Code for Psychologists and Code of Conduct (American Psychological Association, 2002, 2010) serves as the guiding document for the professional behaviors of psychologists, and clearly addresses the issue of the potential impact of the clinician's personal problems on their professional practice:

> **2.06 Personal Problems and Conflicts**
>
> (a) Psychologists refrain from initiating an activity when they know or should know that there is a substantial likelihood that their personal problems will prevent them from performing their work-related activities in a competent manner.

When it is clear that a personal problem may impact your practice, it is probably easier to navigate around the potential pitfalls and avoid ethical problems. However, there are some situations that become problematic once we are already involved.

> (b) When psychologists become aware of personal problems that may interfere with their performing work-related duties adequately, they take appropriate measures, such as obtaining professional consultation or assistance and determine whether they should limit, suspend or terminate their work-related duties.

Some of the most common ethical violations that result in a clinician having their license suspended or revoked involve boundary violations and practicing outside the boundaries of one's area of competence.

2.01 Boundaries of Competence

> (a) Psychologists provide services, teach and conduct research with populations and in areas only within the boundaries of their competence, based on their education, training, supervised experience, consultation, study or professional experience.

In my opinion, these ethical violations occur in part because the clinician, at the beginning of the slippery slope, is not engaged with colleagues such that they can receive feedback and direction that may increase their insight and awareness into their risky thoughts and behaviors, or give them specific recommendations towards the goal of helping to avoid ethical problems.

Whether you are a psychologist, clinical social worker, clinical counselor, or other type of mental health professional, your professional organization undoubtedly has a code of ethics with which you should be familiar. Having an awareness of the ethics we are bound by, and of our duty to practice competently, we should all work harder to engage in practices that will help guide us in the right direction, and to provide a sounding board for our decisions. By sharing dilemmas in a peer consultation, we can check our own thoughts and actions with others who are familiar with the same ethics and guidelines, and ultimately, it can help us make better clinical and ethical decisions.

Nurturing the Caregiver

> Getting feedback and guidance on difficult client cases has helped a great deal in terms of managing feelings of burnout. Having peers who can validate how I feel and help me in maintaining appropriate boundaries with challenging clients has allowed me to feel that I have some "backup" even when I'm in sessions all alone with those clients! I feel that my position and professional opinions on things are clarified and strengthened after discussion in the group. Plus, I often hear suggestions that I hadn't thought of before or that are from different perspectives than my own. — Sara

Take a minute to recall a memory of sitting in a supervision meeting with one of your clinical supervisors during your professional training. How did it feel to admit your uncertainty about how to proceed with a client? What were you thinking when your supervisor asked you questions about your conceptualization or the intervention you implemented? How did you feel at the end of that supervision meeting when you were able to leave feeling supported and given several suggestions to try? Any good supervision experience provides support for the clinician who recognizes their limitations and seeks outside support, guidance, and accountability. Peer consultation can provide the same opportunity to disclose one's uncertainties and receive input and support from colleagues.

Just because supervision may not be required in order to practice once you have achieved your license and independent practice status doesn't mean that it still isn't a good idea. Yes, it can be intimidating to expose your weaknesses to your peers. We don't like to acknowledge that we are stuck with a client or that we don't have all the answers. However, remember that peer consultation is a two-way street—your peer(s) will also be talking about vulnerable areas and seek your guidance as well. We still continue to learn from one another. It's not important that you know all of the answers (no one does), but it is important that you are willing to ask the questions. It's not only a benefit for your client (who reaps the benefit of more professional opinions), it is also an essential and helpful component of the support that you need to sustain yourself as a clinician.

Take a moment to recall a memory of a client with whom you worked, who verbalized feelings of loneliness, isolation, disconnection from others, depression, and frustration. Now think about what you thought would be helpful for them—what recommendations did you offer? One of the things you may have thought of and suggested to your client is that they reconnect with people, build a community, identify, and engage with a group of caring available others. Why are you not taking your own advice? Connecting with other professionals who share similar experiences, frustrations, as well as joys of practice, can be rewarding in so many ways.

Business/Marketing Opportunities

For several years, I went on an annual trip with three colleagues with whom I worked. This trip was work related, but allowed plenty of time for spontaneous conversation about our lives and other professional ventures we were participating in. Invariably, one of us would mention a musing, an idea about some way to provide our professional service or apply our expertise in some new or novel way. It's fun to share ideas with others and listen to their responses. The problem is, most of those ideas were carried home in the minds of the thinker, rarely realized into reality. The outcome might have been different had one of the ideas also been expressed in a consultation group where, not only could the creator of the idea have been asked questions and been given feedback, the idea might have found an opportunity to be tested, or put into practice. One of the challenges of having great ideas as a private practitioner is not just the absence of feedback, but the decreased opportunity to put the idea into action.

Let's say you want to conduct a 6-week, psychoeducational group for adolescent boys who experience depression. Obviously, part of putting a group together means marketing the group and identifying participants—two tasks that could present a challenge if you are not intentionally connected to a group of other professionals. In the context of a consultation group, there would be a ready audience of individuals who, because they know and trust you, would be willing and able to help publicize your group and refer potential participants. You might be thinking, "Well, I could just contact other providers in the area, or send them information about my group." While that is certainly an approach you could take, other providers are less likely to promote and/or refer to someone they do not know and feel that they cannot "vouch" for. By developing these relationships through a peer consultation group, you are providing yourself with an incubator for ideas, allies in developing your ideas, sparks for new concepts or practice options, and a multitude of different ways to engage in the management and clinical work of your practice.

FUN

Since I have shared many practical reasons why a peer consultation group can be beneficial for your clients, for your own feelings of connection, as well as for the good of your practice, it's also important to recognize that peer consultation as a private practitioner has other benefits. It can be fun! Of course, as in any group, you have to get the right people involved, and work to create some group cohesion and a comfort level that can allow group members to move from professional conversations to some of a more personal nature at times. Listen to one peer consultation group member's experiences:

> My current group of 9+ years is certainly my longest standing group. I'm in some other professional groups that are very helpful but not quite the same as our first Thursday of the month group. We talk about LOTS of personal things as well. We've had drinks during group, discussed many milestones in life including marriage, divorce, and parenting, and also have shared tips and secrets about anti-aging procedures. As I am the senior member (chronologically speaking) of our bunch, that information is important!! — A.B.

HOW CAN I MAKE PEER CONSULTATION A PART OF MY PRACTICE?

At this point we know several things. Going into private practice is appealing for many reasons. Those appealing reasons also come with a downside and being a private practitioner brings the risk of isolation, disconnection, and burnout. Although the risk is real, there is a strategy that can mitigate this risk. At first glance it might seem a little daunting to incorporate peer consultation into an already busy life, but I believe it is a valuable self-care practice and well worth your time investment. This next section is intended to help you think about how to integrate peer consultation into your existing and future clinical practice by asking you to reflect on your personal style and your professional needs and wants.

What's My Style? What Am I Looking For?

Creating a peer consultation experience that will be useful and engaging for you will require some assessment of your personal and professional styles as well as an ability to identify what your current needs and desires are. Obviously your needs and desires might change over time (and your peer consultation group may change as well), but you are more likely to consistently participate in a peer consultation experience if you feel that your professional needs are being met in the company of people whom you respect and enjoy spending some time with. There are several questions to ask yourself as you begin thinking about adding peer consultation to your professional life. Thinking about your responses to these questions will not only help you clarify what you need and want, you'll also have a way to assess your experience during your participation, determining how and why peer consultation is or is not working for you. Consider the following:

- Would I prefer a same-sex or coed consultation group?
- Would I prefer all the members in the group to share my theoretical orientation or would I prefer having multiple clinical perspectives?
- How would I feel about the group having an identified "leader?" Would I want to be the "leader/facilitator" of a group?
- How vulnerable am I willing to be? Can I share my uncertainties and areas of discomfort with my peers?
- What's my conflict resolution style? How might I respond if I disagree with something or have strong negative feelings for an issue or an individual in the group?

Now that you have given some thought to the "bigger" questions, we can talk more specifically about the "types" of peer consultation groups there can be. Clearly there is more than one type of peer consultation group; below I have listed several, but the list is not exhaustive, so feel free to use your creativity to come up with your own variation, if one of these doesn't fit your current needs.

As-Needed Consultation

What Is It/What Can It Look Like?

This mode of peer consultation is for clinicians who have identified their need for contact with colleagues but may not be able to commit to a regular schedule and/or have not clarified what their overall "consultation" goals and desires might be. It may consist of a mutual arrangement where you or the other colleague can call one another periodically in order to consult on a particular case. Or perhaps there is something going on in your personal life that might affect your clinical work, and you want some guidance from another professional.

How Could I Establish This?

It would be important to identify one or more available professionals who have a good reputation. You can reach out to them and state what you are looking for and see if they are willing to engage in consultation as needed.

Is This Style of Peer Consultation For Me?

- Do I have limited time to commit to a regular meeting?
- How many other mental health professionals are there in my area with whom to socialize?
- Would I like to have someone to talk to about an ethical dilemma when/if they arise?

Scheduled Socializing with Professional Colleagues

What Is It/What Can It Look Like?

This mode of peer consultation is for clinicians who may not feel they need particular consultation around professional or clinical issues, but desire interaction with colleagues that offers the opportunity to discuss professional matters in a more casual, informal environment.

How Could I Establish This?

You may connect with other professional colleagues through your graduate school, work settings, other colleagues, workshops, or professional organizations. This contact can be casual, and may not require formal arrangements beyond inviting colleagues to go to dinner together, have drinks, or even go bowling. The activity doesn't really matter as long as it is fun and you are able to have the social time you crave. Suggesting a regular rotation (e.g., the third Wednesday of the month) can be a nice way to ease into a scheduled time. Alternately, you could send out emails to assess interest and find out what people like to do together.

Is This Style of Peer Consultation For Me?

- Am I more interested in talking about my personal life than clinical issues?
- Do I already have the clinical support that I need?
- Am I looking to reduce my sense of professional isolation?
- Am I new to the area and want to meet the colleagues around me?

Scheduled Consultation-Professional Agenda

What Is It/What Can It Look Like?

My personal experience of peer consultation has been as a member of a group of five female psychologists who maintain private practices. The group meets 1 day per month for approximately 2 hours to discuss cases, recent changes in managed care, ethical issues, and whatever personal/life issues that might be weighing on us. Having a specific day and time to meet provides structure and allows the members of the group to feel assured that whatever concerns or challenges they might face during the month can be shared with the group.

How Could I Establish This?

How this type of peer consultation comes into existence has no specific formula, but it does require that someone take the initiative to assess the interest of potential members. The potential members could share clinical interests, be from the same part of town, be of the same age cohort, etc. The group could be as homo/heterogeneous as the members prefer, as long as they all agree to meet on a regular basis.

Is This Style of Peer Consultation For Me?

- Do I have the ability to commit to a regular time each month?
- Am I interested in investing in relationships with other professional colleagues to gain different perspectives and share clinical insights?
- Am I interested in receiving feedback from others about my clinical cases even if it's from another theoretical perspective?

Journal Club

What Is It/What Can It Look Like?

During one's graduate training, reading empirical literature was a routine occurrence, but when we enter professional practice, accessing and reading scholarly articles can quickly become a thing of the past. Running the clinical and business sides of a private practice consumes much of our available time, leaving little room in the schedule to seek out and read research that may inform our clinical practice. The issue of time affects those who are new to private practice as well as veterans, but those who have been providing clinical services for a period of time also encounter another potential obstacle—confidence (some might call it arrogance). When you have been engaged in clinical work for a while, you begin to trust yourself, and tend to "do what you've always done," even when research may demonstrate new, empirically informed ways of intervening. One of the ways to ensure that your clinical skills stay sharp and relevant is to engage with colleagues who share your professional and/or clinical interest area around a discussion of current research that informs your practice. Participating in a journal club offers you the chance to interact with peers around a specific topic or subject area without the inherent pressure of socializing. A colleague of mine was in a journal club where the members took turns finding a peer-reviewed journal article of interest and distributing it to the group in advance so everyone could read it. Then they would meet for dinner and discuss the article. As with many group meetings, once the journal discussion had ended, the conversation often drifted into other clinical areas or other social topics.

How Could I Establish This?

Assess the interest of colleagues that you know from professional circles, and ensure that at least one group member has access to journal databases. Many graduate schools allow alumni to access their online library database, which can help with this effort.

Is This Type of Peer Consultation For Me?

- Do I enjoy having a structure and set of expectations for group meetings?
- Do I want to know more about cutting-edge research in order to improve my practice?
- Am I willing/do I have time to locate and read articles to prepare for journal club meetings?

Peer Consultation Via Technology

What Is It/What Can It Look Like

At this time in history it is almost cliché to say that technology affords us so many opportunities to interact with one another; of course it does, and by this point, even those of us who are "digital immigrants" consider ourselves relatively expert in the domain of online social interactions. Using video cameras and videoconferencing tools, or even just a telephone, can make it easy to engage in professional consultation from your office with just about anyone in the world.

How Could I Establish This?

In this approach you are not limited geographically to the connections that you make. Therefore you can keep in touch with clinical mentors, even after you (or they) have moved to another region. You can make connections with experts in the field that you may meet at conferences, or whom you connect with through listservs or other networking websites. The possibilities are endless.

Is This Type of Peer Consultation For Me?

- Do I have mentors or other people who are not near me that I would like to seek consultation from?
- Am I in a geographically isolated or rural area where I do not have the opportunity to connect with other mental health professionals?
- Is there an area of professional practice in which I want additional mentoring with a content expert?

Being a professional helper is often a time-consuming, emotionally taxing experience that also has many professional and personal rewards. When you make the decision to pursue this professional path within a private practice, your experience will likely bring specific opportunities and challenges. Being in private practice has many benefits, including being your own boss, the ability to create a flexible schedule, expanding your income potential, and working with the types of clients and issues you enjoy working with. While these are certainly advantages of being a private practitioner, there are factors that make these benefits potential liabilities. One of the most common liabilities that you will encounter is the isolation that comes from working hard to build and maintain a practice. Isolation from a professional community puts you at risk for burnout, ethical breaches, and disconnection from a professional community who could be a major source of support and encouragement. No matter if you are considering a move into private practice or if you are already working in a practice, there will be times when you will need to step out of your office and engage with others for your personal and professional well-being. Intentionally seeking out other colleagues with whom to spend time and discuss your clinical work allows you the opportunity to expand your clinical skills, feel connected to other professionals in your community, discuss and (hopefully) avoid ethical problems with clients, and develop a group of people to whom you can refer clients and receive client referrals. When you are busy, and focused on building your practice, you may wonder how to get and stay connected to your peers. Stepping into relationships with our peers can be both exciting and daunting, but intention and preparation can make the process a little easier. Preparation includes reflecting on your current needs and wants, and identifying which of the various types of consultation groups works for you. When you find your place amongst your peers, sharing, learning, and consulting with others, you'll find that you feel more connected, more supported, and less isolated; and isn't that a wonderful way to be in your professional life?

REFERENCES

American Psychological Association. (2002). Ethical principles of psychologists and code of conduct. *American Psychologist, 57,* 1060–1073.

American Psychological Association. (2010). 2010 Amendments to the 2002 Ethical Principles of Psychologists and Code of Conduct. *American Psychologist, 65*(5), 493.

Lewis, G.J., Greenburg, S.L., & Hatch, D.B. (1988). Peer consultation groups for psychologists in private practice: A national survey. *Professional Psychology: Research and Practice, 19*(1), 81–86.

SUGGESTED READING

Barry, P. (2006). Forming and belonging to a peer consultation group for your own mental health and creating a psychotherapy practice that addresses specific topics. *Perspectives in Psychiatric Care, 42*(1), 63–66.

Rhodius, A. & Sugarman, K. (2014). Peer consultations with colleagues: The significance of gaining support and avoiding the 'Lone Ranger trap.' In J.G. Cremades, L.S. Tashman, J.G. Cremades, & L.S. Tashman (Eds.), *Becoming a sport, exercise, and performance psychology professional: A global perspective* (pp. 331–338). New York, NY: Psychology Press.

Truneckova, D., Viney, L.L., Maitland, H., & Seaborn, B. (2010). Personal construct peer consultation: Caring for the psychotherapists. *Clinical Supervisor, 29*(2), 128–148.

Chapter 8

Work-life Demands

Practical Tips for Finding the Balance

Emily Sander

In today's fast-paced world, it can be incredibly difficult for individuals to build a rich and fulfilling life, both in and outside of work. Therapists are not exempt from this challenge. Over the past 3 to 4 decades, the concept of work-life balance, or integration, has gathered steam generated from a growing concern that quality of life for individuals is deteriorating in all spheres, including home, work, and community. A simple Google search of *work-life balance* at the time of this writing produced more than 174 million results, ranging from tips for workers on how to achieve it to advice for employers on why to support it; from the benefits of finding it to the consequences of not attaining it. There are countless websites and firms dedicated to helping individuals achieve this complex balance, with promises of fulfillment and greater life satisfaction for those who do. This overabundance of information and resources dedicated to work-life balance illustrates one thing quite clearly; there is a general demand for this elusive state of being.

So, why now? Why has work-life balance become a relevant issue? Many changes in work, culture, and community over the past few decades have influenced the need for greater integration of the work and home spheres. Some of the changes that have influenced the need for improved integration of work and life include advances in technology, changes in the infrastructure of communities, and transitions in individual and societal expectations, such as shifts in gender roles. These changes, and more, that have influenced the call for work-life balance will be discussed throughout this chapter.

At first glance, it may seem that the world of private practice is the ideal setting in which individuals may achieve their ideal balance between work and home roles. It is true that, in many cases, private practice may be exempt from some of the common obstacles to work-life balance, such as employer demands and rigid work schedules. However, many challenges remain that all employed individuals must face, as well as considerations unique to the world of private practice.

The goal of this chapter will be to highlight common challenges to work-life balance faced by mental health professionals, and to help readers identify ways to integrate their work, family, and personal lives in a private practice setting. This chapter will begin by helping individuals to determine what work-life balance means to them through assessment of personal values. Readers will learn how to engage in structured goal setting, with the purpose of developing an action plan for the pursuit of work-life balance. Additionally, this chapter will address psychosocial and logistical issues that may contribute to the perception of balance in the private practice world. Overall, the goal of this chapter will be to help providers in all different stages of career and life identify how to make private practice work for them.

WHAT IS BALANCE?

The term *work-life balance* can be misleading, as the name implies two misassumptions: First, that there should be an equal weight of work outside the home and life outside of work, and second, that "work," "life," and "balance" are simple concepts with shared meanings across all individuals. In reality, there are a wealth of individual factors that affect a person's perception of both the meaning of balance as well as one's perception of personal success in managing work and life in a balanced way. Therefore, it is illogical to presume that there is a standard formula for balance that applies to all. For one, advancement and notoriety in the work world may be a central life interest, thus increasing the desire for, and potential enjoyment drawn from, paid employment outside of the home. For this individual, a sense of satisfaction, or balance, is more likely to be found in greater time, energy, and attention directed at employed work. For another individual, work outside of the home may simply be a means to an end; something one does to support a central life interest of spending time with family, friends, hobbies, or other life pursuits. Neither of these individuals is likely to be satisfied, or feel balanced, in a situation that places equal emphasis on the work and home spheres. In light of these concerns, scholars and lay individuals alike often forgo the term "balance," opting instead for terms like "satisfaction" and "integration." In this chapter, we retain the word "balance," because it is a recognizable concept for many. However, we utilize the label work-life balance to represent the concept of the unique work-life arrangement specific to a given individual that allows for a perceived healthy integration of and personal satisfaction with life, both in and out of the work world.

Work-life balance is not merely about spending equal time invested in work and nonwork pursuits. Rather, it is about feeling a sense of satisfaction with one's entire life (Berry, 2010). It is also not an endpoint or state that can be achieved or completed. Rather, the pursuit of work-life balance is an ongoing process with which one will engage throughout life and career (Berry, 2010). The pursuit of balance is an exercise in how to allocate resources, time, and energy in such a way that one feels fulfilled in day-to-day life, but is also influenced by whether or not the way one spends his or her time matches personal life goals (Berry, 2010).

Contributing Factors to Work-life Imbalance

In order to understand how to best gain, or regain, a desired integration of work and life, it is useful to explore some of the factors that contribute to imbalance. One such contributing factor is the makeup of therapeutic work itself. Therapeutic work is by its very nature, demanding. A therapist's role is to listen to and assist in the alleviation of other people's distress. While not intentional, a therapist may absorb a client's distress, and begin to feel that the work is bleeding into nonwork life. Even the most seasoned therapist is likely to have difficulty separating from the job from time to time.

Another contributing factor to work-life imbalance involves the technological advances of the twenty-first century. Advances in information technology have increased demands on individuals in many fields of employment, and arguably, few are more greatly impacted than the outpatient psychotherapist. Where once there was a distinction between work and home, there is now a blurred boundary. Thanks to advances such as the Internet, smart phones, and home computing, and their impact on the speed of communication, modern therapists must often battle against unrealistic demands on their time and availability. Other factors that can impact imbalance include the demands of managed care and insurance companies, tedium in documentation due to increased demands for liability prevention, environmental factors such as longer average commute times, and financial stresses associated with the escalating costs of education and student loans. In the upcoming pages, we will review factors contributing to burnout in greater detail in order to provide a framework for understanding how to address the problem.

Balance and Burnout

The work of a psychotherapist can be emotionally and mentally taxing due to the nature of the services provided. The role of helping individuals manage life difficulties, often including severe traumas, can lead a caregiver to experience burnout, compassion fatigue, and even vicarious traumatization if the proper care is not taken to prevent this. Burnout has been defined as a state of emotional, physical, psychological, and/or spiritual exhaustion in response to chronic job stressors when working with vulnerable populations (Meichenbaum, 2007). Burnout can lead to disengagement from others and diminished feelings of self-efficacy in the workplace (Meichenbaum, 2007). Compassion fatigue, a term originally introduced by Figley (1995), refers to the fatigue, emotional stress, and potential indifference to the suffering of others that can result from chronic exposure to such suffering or needs expressed by others (Meichenbaum, 2007). Therapists, who often spend their workdays listening to the trials of others, are at greater risk for compassion fatigue than the general population (Meichenbaum, 2007). This increased risk heightens the therapist's need for work-life balance. Similarly, psychotherapists are at risk for vicarious traumatization (VT), which is the cumulative transformation of the inner experience of the therapist that stems from the negative effects of caring for or engaging empathically with and about others and their traumatic material over time (Pearlman & Saakvitne, 1995). Vicarious traumatization is similar to the prior two concepts, but describes a more lasting impact on a provider's sense of self and his or her world (Meichenbaum, 2007).

Compassion fatigue, VT, and burnout can all be indicators of poor work-life balance. Some signs that a provider may be experiencing burnout, compassion fatigue, or VT include feeling overwhelmed or drained, experiencing a loss of pleasure, experiencing feelings of isolation or alienation, preoccupation with thoughts of clients outside of work, questioning of competence, overextending one's self, experiencing difficulties maintaining boundaries with clients, and job dissatisfaction (Meichenbaum, 2007). Job factors that can influence burnout and the like include professional isolation, absence of peer support and supervision, lack of clinical and personal support in the workplace, large caseloads, underutilization of coping skills, excessive time demands, unrealistic expectations of client progress, and low perceived fulfillment of personal and career goals (Meichenbaum, 2007).

Primary methods for preventing and coping with burnout, compassion fatigue, and VT incorporate intentional self-awareness, professional and general self-care, strategic management of work-related activities, and maintenance of social support. Not surprisingly, these are also methods that are useful in the pursuit and maintenance of work-life integration. Later in this chapter, advice on self-care strategies, the benefits of social support, and tips for the management of work-related activities will be explored.

TAKING ACTION

The first, most essential step in creating a satisfying integration, or balance, of work and life is to assess what you actually want—and need—out of life as a whole. After all, it is very difficult to head in the right direction if you do not know the destination in the first place. One useful method in determining what you want and need from life is to engage in a values assessment, an example of which we will practice later in this chapter. Once you have a clear picture of what you are looking for, the next step is to determine short- and long-term goals directed at the pursuit of balance. Lastly, you must determine periodic assessment time points, at which you will reevaluate goals and adjust plans accordingly. The final step is necessary, as work-life balance is not a static target. After all, what you want and need from life will evolve over time; therefore, it is important to reassess work-life satisfaction and long-term goals from time to time.

Determining Values and Setting Goals

Goal setting is more than merely stating the desire for something to happen. It is a strategic method of identifying and defining exactly what you want and the steps necessary to achieve those goals. When individuals feel that they are not heading anywhere in life, or that they are not heading in the direction that they want to go, it is likely that they have not spent enough time considering what it is, exactly, they want from life (their values), and have not set clear goals for themselves. Not only does goal setting help define a path; it also helps spark motivation to make what may have once been ambiguous goals into an achievable reality. Further, once goals are clearly defined, there is a better understanding of how to organize time and allocate resources. By engaging in a structured goal-setting process, your odds of successful goal achievement are considerably improved. Here, we will illustrate a four-step goal-setting process to guide you in the pursuit of work-life balance.

Goal Setting Step 1: Know Thy Self

Begin the goal-setting process by identifying the large-scale goals that you would like to achieve, either in a lifetime, or in a designated period of time, such as 10 to 15 years. Setting lifetime goals is the initial step, because it helps to give direction to the remainder of the planning process. It is important that lifetime goals be identified for all significant areas of your life in order to maintain focus on finding balance. To help guide the identification of lifetime goals, it is useful to look at personal values. Personal values are your convictions about what you believe to be important and desirable. Personal values can be either terminal, meaning they are desired end-states you hope to reach, or instrumental, meaning desired traits with which you wish to be associated. Terminal values, or goals, are things like becoming "a good parent" or "a successful psychologist," while instrumental values include adjectives like developing "assertiveness" and "creativity." In this chapter we will focus on the more concrete terminal values.

Individuals can value many things at once; therefore, it is possible for personal values to come into conflict with one another. For instance, an individual's family value of being a stay-at-home parent during the early childhood years may be in conflict with a career value of achieving a certain level of distinction within the academic field by a certain age. When such conflicts arise, they can be resolved through value prioritization. Understanding values helps increase self-awareness, which ultimately allows for identification of what about themselves or their choices individuals want or need to change (Whetten & Cameron, 2002). When you examine how well current choices fit with values, you are better able to make appropriate adjustments, avoid choices that are guided by impulse or instant gratification, and improve time management.

The list below is representative of common categories in which personal values may be identified. These categories are not exhaustive, and can be added to as desired.

- Family
- Personal development
- Education/knowledge
- Career
- Religious/spiritual
- Health/physical
- Contribution/service
- Creative
- Enjoyment/hobby
- Travel
- Financial

For each of these categories, list personal values and any related goals you would like to achieve over the course of your lifetime. For instance, a *value* in the "family category" may be prioritizing family time, while family-oriented *goals* may be to have children, to be able to attend all of a child's activities, to care for an aging parent, and so on. A career *value* may be to do work that is spiritually fulfilling, while career *goals* may include gaining a desired level of distinction in the field, specific publication goals, development of a certain specialty, or to work for a certain program or institution. In order to better explore these values and goals, you can ask yourself the following questions for each of the categories listed above:

- What are the most important achievements for me in this category?
- How will I know I have reached my desired goal(s)?
- Do other goals or values depend on achievements in this category?
- What things in this category, if not completed in my lifetime, will lead to disappointment? In the next 15 years? In the next 5 years? In the next year?

Once you have determined your lifetime goals, rank them in order of priority. It may be useful to concentrate on the top three or four goals on this list, as addressing too many goals at once can become overwhelming and difficult to organize. During this process it is important to reflect on whether or not the items identified are truly goals that you personally want to achieve, rather than choices that are influenced by what others want. It is easy to be influenced by what those around us, such as parents, spouses, employers, peers, or even society at large view as priorities. While it is okay to consider others, particularly spouses, in the goal-identification process, ultimately, a personal sense of balance cannot be achieved if you are not addressing personal desires.

Goal Setting Step 2: Go For the Goals

The next step is to break your lifetime goals down into progressively smaller goals, representing the various targets you must hit in order to achieve life-time goals. For instance, you may choose to complete a 10-year plan, 5-year plan, 1-year plan, 6-month plan, and/or a 1-month plan. Each successive plan should be based upon the prior plan. For instance, if one large-scale goal is to write a book, some stepping-stone goals might include attending continuing education courses on topics of interest, writing specific book chapters, documenting case studies related to the topic area, networking with publishers, or seeking advice from other professionals who have achieved similar goals. Breaking these examples down into some progressive goals may look something like this:

Two-year plan:

- Be under contract with a publisher
- Have a draft of the full manuscript ready for editing

One-year plan:

- Schedule or attend at least two continuing education courses on the identified book topic
- Reach out to publishing houses to investigate interest
- Have at least two book chapters in draft form to submit to potential publishers

Six-month plan:

- Have a book topic identified
- Speak to at least two peers who have been published about their experiences and recommendations
- Begin to document all case studies relevant to the book topic
- Seek release of information/permission from any clients whose case studies may be useful in book writing

One month plan:

- Make a list of interest areas and/or areas of expertise about which you may want to write
- Do an Internet and/or library search to explore demand and/or need for texts on the identified topics
- Look into continuing education programs available in relation to potential book topics
- Complete an Internet and library search for publishing houses that publish texts in this category

Setting S.M.A.R.T. Goals

In order to develop the tiered plans in the above-mentioned process, it is useful to have a guide for goal setting. For the past several decades, the business world has used the mnemonic S.M.A.R.T. to describe key elements of effective goal setting. There are numerous variations of the S.M.A.R.T. mnemonic, but for the purposes of this exercise it stands for setting Specific, Measureable, Attainable, Relevant, and Time-bound goals. While S.M.A.R.T. was developed with the management and business world in mind, it is also an effective tool in personal goal development.

S—Specific

Specific or precise goals are more likely to be accomplished than vague or overly broad goals because they are clear and leave little room for doubt about what is expected. For example, a goal of "eating healthier" is far more vague and lacking in direction than the goal of "purchase a healthy eating cookbook and, as a family, cook one new recipe at home each week to increase family time and healthy eating." A specific goal has a much greater chance of being accomplished than a general goal because it tells the person exactly what is expected and why. One way to make a goal more specific is to define what terms within the goal mean. In the previous example, you would explore how you define "healthier" eating in order to identify more specific objectives. In this case, more specific goals might be to reduce calorie intake to a certain number, to reduce intake of processed foods, or to eliminate alcohol consumption. A helpful method in developing specific goals is to utilize the five Ws: who, what, when, where, and why.

Who: Identify who is involved and can be supportive or helpful in achieving your goal.

What: Establish what you want to accomplish.

When: Establish a time frame or deadline.

Where: Identify a location.

Why: Specify why you are trying to accomplish this goal. What are the reasons, purpose, or benefits of accomplishing the goal?

Tip: State each goal in positive, performance-oriented terms, rather than negative, outcome-oriented terms (e.g., "Be physically active at least 30 minutes each day," rather than "Don't gain weight"). Outcomes are not always based upon things within your control, but effort, or performance, is. Writing positively worded goals allows you to focus on what you want, rather than on what you want to avoid.

M—Measurable (Meaningful, or Motivating)

It can be quite difficult to know if you are making progress toward a goal if there is no established way to measure progress. By establishing concrete criteria for measuring progress toward each goal, standards for success can be identified. Further, measureable goals allow you to know how far you have come and how much further you must go, allowing you to stay on track.

Measurable goals are often numbers based, or quantitative, but they can also be descriptive. Quantitative goals are the easiest to track and measure, and are therefore ideal. An example of a quantitative goal for writing a manuscript would be, "Have 200 pages written by March 1st." A descriptive goal is one that clearly describes the desired outcome so that it is easily recognizable when it has been achieved. For example, a descriptive goal for writing a manuscript would be, "Have completed document approved by an editor by March 1st."

Some questions you might ask yourself in order to determine if a goal is measurable include:

- How will I know when it is accomplished?
- How many? (e.g., How many pages do I want to have completed by my deadline?)
- How much? (e.g., How much time do I need to accomplish the goal?)
- What will it look like when I have achieved the goal?

Tip: Write goals down. This creates a set of instructions for both the conscious and subconscious mind to carry out. When we engage in the act of writing down goals, it makes them more real or concrete in our mind's eye.

A—Attainable

The third step in S.M.A.R.T. goal identification is to determine if the goals established are attainable, or realistic. An attainable goal is one toward which you are both willing and able to work. The greatest risk in forgetting to assess the attainability of a goal is that of becoming discouraged. If you set the bar too high, you will invariably become discouraged when either progress toward the goal is too slow or when the realization hits that the goal is unlikely to be achieved. By taking care to make sure goals are attainable from the outset, you can avoid such pitfalls. To be clear, being attainable does not mean that a goal cannot be ambitious; it merely means that it must be possible to achieve with the proper resources.

In order to create attainable goals, it is useful to consider any foreseeable barriers that might stand in the way of completion, as well as potential means to overcome them. While there will be challenges to face on the path to any goal, one must determine the feasibility of overcoming the predicted challenges. For instance, if you set a goal of being elected to a state licensing board within 2 years of licensure, you would be setting yourself up for disappointment if you are licensed in one of the many states that requires at least 3 years of licensure to be considered for such a role. This is a barrier that one is highly unlikely to overcome. In this case, the time frame of the goal could be adjusted to make the goal more attainable.

While assessing attainability, it is a good time to self-reflect upon any limitations that may interfere with success, including personal limitations. If, upon reflection, you do not think you can realistically achieve the goal without dramatic changes to your current life or personality, it is best to adjust the goal to something more attainable. Keep in mind, a long-term goal can be realistic even if you do not currently have the proper resources to achieve it, as long as a plan for the acquisition of necessary resources is an element of the goal-completion process.

To examine attainability, you may ask yourself the following:

- How much time do I have to dedicate to my goal (and how much time is it likely to require)? For example, if work, family, and social life leave you with only an hour of free time each day, a goal of training for a marathon in less than a year's time is fairly unrealistic.
- What personal limitations may impact my ability to follow-through on or achieve my goal? For example, does your tendency toward procrastination impact the likelihood of working on a certain goal a little each day? Or, does having a physical limitation impact the manner in which your goal may be achieved?
- What external limitations may impact my ability to follow-through on or achieve my goal? For example, how realistic is it to have a goal of having children by a certain age if you are currently without a partner, a factor over which you may have limited control?
- What financial limitations may impact my ability to achieve my goal? For example, is it realistic to plan to buy a house within the next year if you currently have significant debt?
- What are the roles in my life, and how do they conflict with and benefit each other? For example, does being a parent, a caregiver to an aging parent, or a student interact in some way with the ability to engage in therapeutic practice?

There are few goals that cannot be obtained with the proper preparation and right attitude. Trouble shooting barriers before they arise is not an exercise in focusing on the negative; rather, it is a way of charting the course so that the negative is avoided. Once the potential barriers are addressed, the path to your goals is clearer, and you can begin to see that your goals are within reach.

In addition to assessing the feasibility of a goal, it is also useful to evaluate your personal level of commitment to the goal and the plan through which it will be achieved. To determine the level of commitment, ask yourself questions such as:

- Do I feel committed, at present, to the steps I have outlined to reach my goal?
- Am I willing to make the necessary alterations to my life outlined in my plan?
- Am I committed to giving the time needed to complete the goal, even if it takes away from other aspects of my life?

If you answer no to these questions, it may be best to reconsider your targets, and adjust them accordingly. It is challenging to achieve a goal if the goal and your level of commitment to it do not correspond. For instance, if your goal is to write a book over the course of a 2-year period, but you are unwilling to cut into family time in order to have time to write, then you will likely need to adjust your expectations.

Tips:

- Ambitious goals can often be easier to reach than mundane ones, because they are more likely to spark motivation.
- When setting goals, it is essential to be honest with yourself about the changes and efforts you are willing to make, otherwise you may set the stage for failure.

R—Relevant

Relevant, according to Google (2016), is defined as being "closely connected or appropriate to the matter at hand." When it comes to goal setting, the matter at hand is the individual and his or her desires. Therefore, relevant goals are goals that matter to *you*, not goals that matter to other people. If the goals set are based upon expectations others have, or on external priorities, you are unlikely to feel motivated to achieve them—or satisfied if you do. After all, if a person does not really want something, then why would they bother to work hard to get it? If a goal is relevant to your personal desires then it should, by its very nature, be intrinsically rewarding. If the goal you have set does not feel like a reward for all the hard work it will take to achieve it, then it may be time to question if it is really a relevant goal.

During this process, do not forget to explore how various goals and plans to achieve them fit with one another. For example, if your plan to achieve career goals conflicts with plans to achieve family goals, one or both plans will likely require adjustment.

Suggested questions to ask yourself when assessing relevance are:

- Why do I want to achieve this goal?
- Are these goals unduly influenced by outside opinions or expectations?
- Do these goals make me feel energized and excited? How so?
- In what way do I think I will feel fulfilled if I achieve this goal?
- Will the work needed to achieve my goals feel like a burden?

Tip: When you have several goals, which you should when working towards work-life balance, assign a priority to each. This will help you identify when and where to direct your attention.

T—Time-bound (Trackable, or Tangible)

A time-bound goal is one that has a deadline or a time frame within which it is to be completed. The benefit of deadlines is that they create a sense of urgency, thereby increasing motivation to work toward goal completion. By imposing time frames upon the plans, one stands a greater chance of following through on the specific actions identified for a given goal.

It is not only important to set a deadline for ultimate goal completion, it is also important to identify benchmarks or time-points for the successful completion of smaller goals. By breaking large goals into small chunks, you can better measure progress. Furthermore, benchmarks provide increased opportunities for success, and thus increased opportunity for reinforcement, which ultimately impacts motivation.

Tips:

- As you address benchmarks on the path to your goals, check in at regularly scheduled intervals to make sure you are still on the path to your long-term goals.
- Tie rewards or incentives to your identified benchmarks to help increase motivation and follow-through.

Goal Setting Step 3: To-do, Today

Finding a desirable balance, or integration, of work and life requires daily effort. In light of this, the next step in goal setting is to establish daily goals or tasks. Some of these tasks will be routine, such as completing treatment notes by a specific time each day. Others will be unique tasks added to a daily to-do list, such as attending a seminar or making a specific contact. The daily to-do list is the one portion of the goal-setting plan that should be updated repeatedly, to make sure that goals are being addressed on a consistent basis.

The daily to-do list will be composed of two parts, the Master List and the Flex List. The Master List is composed of ongoing tasks that one commits to doing everyday in order to make steady progress toward goals. Items on the Master List may include actions like doing 5 minutes of relaxation training, completing treatment notes at a specified time, or reading for a designated period of time daily. Items on the Master List can be directed at gradually achieving large, but time-limited goals, such as completing a manuscript, or on open-ended goals, such as reducing stress levels over time. The Flex List is composed of distinct tasks that are intended to be completed in a few sittings or less, such as conducting a specific Internet search, attending a course, or going to a doctor's appointment. By documenting and completing both types of daily tasks, you can remain on track with broader personal goals.

Tips:

- As you begin to address your goals, you will realize that it takes considerable energy. It is useful to think about and begin to eliminate the things in your daily life that take time and energy away from your priorities. Make a conscious effort to eliminate or reduce time-wasting or disadvantageous activities.
- If you feel overwhelmed, begin small. Improving balance does not necessarily require dramatic alterations to your routine. Even small changes can make a notable difference in your quality of life.

Goal Setting Step 4: Reward, Review, Repeat

Goal setting and achievement is hard work, so when a goal is reached, whether it be a smaller benchmark or a larger lifetime accomplishment, it is wise to take the time to honor your success. Revel in the satisfaction of having accomplished something you set out to do. When you achieve a significant goal, or a goal that was particularly strenuous to reach, it is beneficial to reward yourself in some tangible way. Without reward there is little motivation to press forward.

Once you have rewarded yourself for your accomplishments, review the remaining goals and make updates and adjustments as necessary. When a task is completed, add another action step to replace it to keep moving forward. Keep in mind that goal setting is an ongoing, fluid activity, and as such, goals and plans may need to be altered from time-to-time. In order to monitor the need for adjustments to goals, it is a good idea to build in regularly scheduled review points at which goals are examined and adjusted. Even when lifetime goals remain the same over time, the steps necessary to achieve these goals may require alteration based upon fluctuations in life circumstances, priorities, or resources. Scheduling check-points can prevent following a dead-end path and can also allow for adjustments to goals based upon any difficulties that may arise. For instance, if a benchmark goal is taking exceptionally long to achieve, a check-in can bring this to light and provide the opportunity to break the goal down into smaller, more manageable parts. Conversely, if ongoing goals are being achieved with excessive ease, checkpoints afford the opportunity to recognize this and adjust those goals to be appropriately challenging.

Tips:

- Remind yourself regularly of the progress you have made and how far you have come.
- As you go through your day and are faced with decisions, ask yourself, "Will this decision help me get closer to or farther from my goals?" When your answer is "closer," then you can feel confident moving in that direction. If, however, the answer is "farther," you may want to reconsider the decision you are about to make.

PRACTICAL CONCERNS WITHIN A PRIVATE PRACTICE SETTING

Now that goals have been identified and an action plan created, it is time to explore practical concerns that can impact work-life balance in the private practice world. It has become increasingly uncommon for individuals today to seek distinct separation of work and nonwork life. Rather, emphasis has been placed on blending the work and nonwork worlds in a personally satisfying way. The following explores common challenges to this blend that are particularly relevant to private practice. Suggestions are made to help practitioners navigate such challenges.

Technology and Boundaries

Technological advances of the twenty-first century have intensified demands for treatment providers' time and have increased overlap of home and work roles. Where once there was a clear distinction between work and home, there is now a blurred boundary with seemingly endless demands for providers' time. Once upon a time, a provider's obligation to clients was to be available in person during treatment sessions and possibly by phone in emergency situations. The Internet, smart phones, voicemail, and home computing have shifted the modern expectation for provider accessibility towards a demand for constant availability with pressure to be perpetually "at the ready" to address client needs. The combination of email and smart phones effectively enables a client to send a message directly to a provider's pocket at any given time of the day. It is more difficult than ever before to unplug from work. This leaves the provider with decisions regarding what boundaries to institute with clients and other work contacts, so that work does not perpetually invade home life.

As previously mentioned, it is unlikely in most scenarios that a provider will be able to, or perhaps even desire to, have a complete separation between work and home spheres. For example, there are certainly benefits of being able to check voice and electronic mail remotely, at times of the provider's choosing, rather than to be tethered to the office. However, if no boundaries are put in place with these remote connections, a provider can easily slip into the trap of being at clients' beck and call. In order for you to determine the best boundaries for your situation, you may begin by asking yourself the following questions:

- What are my "do not disturb" moments in life?
- What are my obligations to the population I serve?
- What are my personal views about turn-around time for client and professional requests?
- What are the requirements of my particular licensing body and any insurance providers with whom I contract?

Example:

Dr. Parent is a married guardian of three young children whose client population is predominantly adolescents and young adults. Dr. Parent identifies "do not disturb" times as any time between the hours of 5:00PM and 9:00PM on weekdays, during which dedicated family time is prioritized. Therapist off days and holidays are also considered "do not disturb" times. Many of Dr. Parent's clients are being treated for high-need or high-risk issues, such as personality disorders and disordered eating. The nature of these issues increases the need for clear boundaries, but also increases the likelihood of the clients reaching out to the therapist between sessions. Because this is a particularly vulnerable population, Dr. Parent feels committed to checking for client messages at least once daily, even on off days. Dr. Parent's personal views are that client contacts should be acknowledged within a 24-hour period, but that more-detailed responses can be delayed until designated office or documentation hours, or ideally, addressed during client session time. Dr. Parent is licensed in a state that does not have specific regulations regarding therapist availability to clients outside of session times, but is contracted with insurance carriers that require providers to be available in case of emergency.

Based on the results of these questions, Dr. Parent develops the following plan:

In the intake paperwork, Dr. Parent includes a document clearly stating regularly scheduled office hours, as well as personal policies for electronic and telecommunication with clients. This document is reviewed with the client at intake, and all clients must endorse agreement with therapist policies with their signature, establishing this as a contract between client and therapist. The document states that Dr. Parent will make every effort to acknowledge client emails within 24 hours of receipt, but that detailed responses will be reserved for therapist documentation time or addressed in the client's next scheduled session. It is clearly stated that Dr. Parent's daily documentation time is reserved for 10 PM on weeknights and at the therapist's discretion on therapist off days. It is also stated in this document that voicemails left on the office phone will be returned within 48 hours of receipt, but that messages are only checked when the therapist is in the office, which could delay response time. Dr. Parent utilizes an emergency voicemail paging system for emergency calls. This is clearly explained in the intake document, and clients are informed that the therapist's standard voicemail, as well as electronic mail, are not to be utilized in emergency situations. In addition to documenting these details in the intake paperwork, Dr. Parent reiterates these boundaries in the standard voicemail away message and an electronic mail automated reply.

Voicemail message example:

You have reached the voicemail of Dr. A. Parent. Dr. A. Parent is away from the office at this time. Office hours are Monday through Friday, 9 AM through 5 PM. Please be advised that this voicemail box is unattended during the times when Dr. A. Parent is out of the office. Please leave your name, contact information, and a brief message and Dr. A. Parent will return your call within 48 hours of receipt. If you are in crisis, please utilize the emergency paging system. If this is an emergency, please go to the nearest emergency room or call 911.

Automated email reply example:

Your message has been received by Dr. A. Parent, licensed clinical psychologist at Friendly Psychological Services. Dr. A. Parent values your inquiry and will make every effort to respond in a timely manner within 48 hours. Please be advised that Dr. A. Parent is in the office the following days and times, which may impact the timing of the reply to your inquiry:

Mondays: 1 PM to 9 PM
Tuesdays: 9 AM to 5 PM
Wednesdays: Out of office
Thursdays: 1 PM to 9 PM

Fridays: 9 AM to 5 PM
Saturdays: Out of office
Sundays: Out of office

By setting very clear boundaries, such as those illustrated in the previous vignette, a provider can protect personal time without fear of neglecting professional duties. While this method is labor intensive on the front end, it ultimately saves time and confusion for both therapist and clients.

Scheduling Issues

Flexible Scheduling: Thinking Outside of the Monday Through Friday, 9 to 5, Box

One of the central factors that influences perceived work-life balance is perceived job flexibility through methods such as flex time, telecommuting, and nontraditional work schedules (Byrne, 2005; Hill, Hawkins, Ferris, & Weitzman, 2001). Numerous studies have identified that the primary factor employers can address to give workers an increased sense of work-life satisfaction is to offer flexible scheduling options (Guest, 2002; Hill, Hawkins, Ferris, & Weitzman, 2001; Smith & Gardner, 2007). As you might expect, the ability to set one's own schedule is a perk of working in a private practice setting. Some factors worth considering when setting a work schedule include the hours and days in direct contact with clients, time spent on nonface-to-face tasks, how time is managed during hours worked, and the ability to adjust schedules as needed.

The theoretical benefit of flexible scheduling is that you may adapt your work schedule to fit with the demands of home and life. A flexible schedule allows you to work around variables like spouse work schedules, children's school or childcare needs, time demands from other employment, medical and other personal appointments, and other personal factors. However, personal factors are not the only variables that are beneficial to consider when planning a clinical schedule. It is particularly beneficial to take into consideration the needs of the population served when establishing clinical hours and appointment scheduling. Do you treat predominantly school-aged children? Then family-friendly evening and weekend hours will likely be better received, and thus keep business steady. Do you run a geropsychology practice? Then, traditional 9 AM to 5 PM clinic hours may be preferred over evening hours. Or, do you see a range of individuals with diverse needs? If so, then perhaps more diverse clinic hours are in order. Keeping a client-friendly schedule can be key to keeping a steady client flow, and thus, a viable practice.

In phase one of developing a clinic schedule, you can ask yourself the following questions:

- What personal life factors do I need to work around, based upon my priorities?
- What personal life factors would I like to work around?
- What are the needs of the population I serve?
- What am I unwilling to compromise?

Once you have determined the answers to these questions, consider:

- How many clients do I want/need to see in an average week to achieve my desired income?
- How many appointments and total hours a week, on average, are needed to see this number of clients?
- What time slots (days and hours) are most desirable to the population I serve, and thus most likely to draw in steady business?
- How many hours a day do I prefer to work? Do I prefer to work more days with shorter hours, or fewer days with longer hours?
- At what pace do I want to work? Am I okay seeing clients back-to-back, or do I want breaks in between clients?
- Do I want to see a higher average number of clients during busy times of the year, in order to create a financial cushion to supplement reduced income during lighter times of the year? Or do I want to keep the same schedule year-round?

Documentation and Noncontact Hours

In addition to scheduling direct contact hours, individuals who work in a private practice setting must consider how they want to manage scheduling concerns such as documentation time. A provider must consider how to manage completion of progress notes, letter and report writing, electronic mail and voicemail contact, insurance and billing tasks, and the like. There are two primary factors related to task completion that are likely to impact perceptions of work-life balance: fit with personal priorities, and efficiency. For example, for a provider who prioritizes family time, it may be most desirable to restrict clinic time to face-to-face interactions and to complete other functions, such as documentation, from home, thereby allowing the provider to spend as little time away from home as possible. Conversely, for a provider who values distinct separation of the work and home spheres, but who also wants to have as much home time as possible, efficiency is a greater priority. This individual may choose to build documentation time into the daily clinic schedule, so that, though the work day may be longer, by the end of the clinic day the work is finished. You must determine for yourself whether efficiency or fit with personal priorities is of greatest importance based on your situation. In the world of private practice, the key with scheduling is to think outside of the box.

Questions to ask yourself in regard to scheduling of noncontact hours include:

- What are my priorities in terms of how and where my time is spent?
- Where do I do my best work in terms of documentation?
- What time of day do I do my best work in terms of documentation?
- What barriers exist to completing documentation in the home setting? In the office setting?
- Is there a potential financial impact of completing documentation in one location versus the other (such as cost of remote access to electronic medical record software, cost of childcare if away from home, etc.)?
- Are there any potential ethical barriers to completing documentation outside of the office?

Parents of young children, such as Dr. A. Parent from the previous example, may prioritize being home with their children during their waking hours, and thus may choose to do documentation from home after the children have gone to bed. This may be less efficient, but meets the goal of prioritizing family time. A provider without dependent family members, who prioritizes free time in the evenings, may choose to stay at the office until all documentation is completed each day, so that evenings can remain free for nonwork pursuits. This is likely more efficient and meets the provider's personal preferences.

Daily Scheduling Considerations

When developing a clinical schedule, it is not only important to manage the days and times worked, but also to manage the types of clients treated on a given day. A key contributor to therapist burnout is overexposure to client distress. As most clinicians know, clients with certain diagnoses and trauma histories are more emotionally taxing to treat than others. In light of this, it is best to maintain a diversified caseload that includes both high-demand and lower-demand clients and clinical presentations. Where possible, it is advisable to balance your daily schedule so that more intense clients are not seen in close succession. Research has indicated that it is not advisable for providers to spend more than 60 percent of their clinical time working with trauma survivors, so as to reduce likelihood of vicarious traumatization (Taylor, 2006). When developing a caseload, one might ask oneself the following questions:

- Which clinical presentations do I find most emotionally taxing?
- How many clients of a particular presentation or of a high degree of need do I believe I can comfortably treat in a given week? In a given day?

Social and Emotional Concerns

Despite your best efforts to establish a balanced caseload and work schedule, there will be times when the stresses inherent in being a care provider begin to negatively impact your life and mental health. As this stress increases, you may begin to experience feelings of imbalance, or poor integration of work and life demands. In order to prevent and/or address this, providers must engage in stress management behaviors, such as self-care and seeking of social support.

Self-Care

Self-care is a broad term that generally encompasses any intentional actions one may take to care for one's own physical, mental, and emotional health. Professional self-care expands upon this concept, and involves the utilization of strategies and skills to address and maintain one's own needs while continuing to support the needs of the clients one serves (Newell & MacNeil, 2010). Research has shown that engagement in physical and emotional self-care can positively influence an individual's perception of work-life balance, as well as contribute to improved quality of life (Pope & Vasquez, 2005). Professional self-care behaviors that are particularly useful for maintenance of work-life balance involve frequently practiced, low time demand skills, such as practicing relaxation exercises between clients, and engaging in transitional exercises when leaving work.

General behavioral strategies used to combat depression and other mental health concerns, such as maintaining physical fitness, obtaining balanced nutrition, getting adequate sleep, and engaging in recreational activities also serve to buffer the effects of burnout and conditions like it (Newell & MacNeil, 2010). Recreational activities that can be used as an outlet for emotional release include journaling, gardening, and artistic pursuits (Hesse, 2002). Undue emphasis should not be placed on the specifics of the recreational self-care activity with which one chooses to engage. Research indicates that the specifics of a self-care activity are of limited importance, as long as the activity allows for engagement in something that is positive and has concrete outcomes to foster a sense of accomplishment (Meichenbaum, 2007).

Ten self-care strategies for work-life balance have been provided below, as an introduction to seeking balance through preventative self-care. For a more in-depth discussion of self-care and suggested self-care methods, see the Chapter 9 entitled: "Twenty-five Strategies for Engaging in Self-care."

TEN SELF-CARE STRATEGIES FOR WORK-LIFE BALANCE

1. Develop a transition ritual that can be utilized at the end of each workday. The goal is to help trigger the mental transition from work to home. By doing the same ritual at the end of each workday, you condition your brain to associate the ritual with mentally leaving work and its concerns behind.
2. Schedule multiple minibreaks each workday, during which you can engage in brief self-care activities such as diaphragmatic breathing, self-massage, yoga, meditation, eating a snack, text messaging loved ones, or any other activity that allows for relaxation.
3. Avoid excessive delaying of gratification. Stop thinking things like, "Things will be better when…" or "I'll have more time after I finish…" Instead, if you are feeling stressed, focus on what you can do in the moment to improve some aspect of your situation.
4. Use commute time wisely. The drive to and from work is a great time to engage in activities you may otherwise have difficulty fitting into the day, and provides a suitable transition from work to home. Engage in relaxation activities like meditation or deep breathing, listen to audio books, learn a language, listen to mood-boosting music, sing, etc.
5. Dedicate time to one enjoyable activity that requires an external commitment. Having a commitment to someone or something external will increase the odds of follow through on at least that one self-care activity. Join a recreational sports team, take an art class, join a parent's group, join a peer consultation group, etc.
6. Implement routines. Each decision a person makes, no matter how small, takes energy and willpower. Routines reduce the need for decision making on a daily basis. Eliminate rushing in the morning

by creating a structured, nonhurried morning routine. Unwind for sleep by following a consistent bedtime routine.

7. Simplify. If something is not important, eliminate it. Again, each decision you make depletes energy. You can reduce the need for decision making by eliminating decisions that don't matter to you. Don't care about fashion? Create a personal uniform so that less energy goes into thinking about what to wear each day. Feel exhausted by choosing what to do for dinner each night? Implement Meatloaf Mondays and Takeout Tuesdays.
8. Make dates for the important things in your life, including time with kids, friends, your spouse or partner, mentors, etc. If you do not schedule it, it is less likely to happen.
9. Do not be afraid to say "no." Knowing one's limitations, including when one has reached maximum capacity for the demands of work, family, and life, is not a sign of weakness. If your schedule is full, recognize that it is okay to say "no" and take a break.
10. Do not try to be a superhero. Accept that you are not going to be at your best all the time or able to accomplish all that you want to do everyday. If your emotions are telling you that you are overwhelmed, it's a good time to take a step back and let someone help you for a change.

Seeking Support

A key step in maintaining balance between work and life is the utilization of social support. For practicing psychologists, as well as other clinicians, the combination of working in isolation and the task of managing other's emotional difficulties can lead to emotional stress (APA Practice Organization, 2015; Stamm, 1999). This is particularly true when a therapist must manage more intense client concerns (Stamm, 1999). Research suggests a correlation between the perception of social support and reduced work-life stress, or imbalance (Quick, Tetrick, Adkins, & Klunder, 2003).

Substantial evidence suggests that support from professional colleagues and supervisors, in particular, may serve to decrease the effects of professional burnout (Lakey & Cohen, 2000; Ray & Miller, 1994). Support from peers in the field is helpful because peers are more likely to relate to the struggles of being a care provider and the experience of concepts such as burnout and compassion fatigue.

Professional social support can take many forms, including mentorship, peer consultation groups, and utilization of personal psychotherapy.

Individual psychotherapy, in particular, can be a useful tool for the management and prevention of burnout and vicarious traumatization for providers who have experienced trauma or other distress in their personal lives (Nelson-Gardell & Harris, 2003; Hesse, 2002). Another avenue for gaining professional social support is to join a group practice, where one tends to maintain the perks of independence, while benefiting from sharing expenses and avoiding isolation.

A connection to nonwork family, friends, and groups can be another avenue for social support, and thus, improved work-life integration. One role that social support can play for the psychotherapist is in providing a sense of connection to others and to something greater than themselves. Such a connection can be found through engagement with support groups, clubs, religious groups, and other organizations. Emotional and social connections with friends and family has been shown to provide a useful defense against the symptoms of burnout and vicarious traumatization (Figley & Barnes, 2005; Phipps & Burne, 2003). It is not necessary that a connection with others be focused on giving and receiving support. Rather, sharing in enjoyable social activities and trying new experiences with others also serves as a buffer against burnout. Involvement in social activism and charitable contributions can play similarly protective roles.

For greater detail regarding methods of social support, including mentorship, please explore Chapter 7 entitled "Isolation, Disconnection, and Burnout: The Importance of Staying Connected in Private Practice."

IN CLOSING

At first glance, the notion of achieving a satisfying integration, or balance, of work and life may not seem like a difficult task for a mental health clinician to achieve. After all, few people make the choice to become care providers without an underlying sense of passion and dedication to helping others, and, in theory, a career based on passion ought to be satisfying. But, as discussed above, even when you truly enjoy your career, a variety of variables, both in- and outside of your control, can develop into obstacles on the path to balance. After completing the exercises in this chapter, you will be better able to both identify what will give you a sense of balance in life and career and be able to construct a pathway to achieve that balance through goal setting. Once the path to balance is constructed, you will be better prepared to recognize when something interrupts your sense of work-life balance and be more prepared to restore that balance through corrective action. On the pathway to your goals, you may not feel the "balance" everyday, but you will hopefully feel greater satisfaction and stability overall, and when it comes to balance, that's what it's all about.

REFERENCES

APA Practice Organization (n.d). Health and well-being for psychologists. Retrieved ON 10/13/2015 from http://www.apapracticecentral.org/ce/self-care/well-being.aspx.

Berry, E. (2010). Achieving work-life balance: More than just a juggling act. *American Medical News*. Retrieved from http://www.amednews.com/article/20100104/business/301049968/4/.

Byrne, U. (2005). Work-life balance: Why are we talking about it at all? *Business Information Review, 22*(1), 53–59.

Figley, C.R. (1995). Compassion fatigue: Toward a new understanding of the costs of caring. In B.H. Stamm (ed). (1995). *Secondary traumatic stress: Self-care issues for clinicians, researchers, and educators,* (pp. 3–28). Baltimore, MD: The Sidran Press.

Figley, C.R. & Barnes, M.F. (2005). External Trauma and families. In P.C. McKenry & S.J. Price (Eds.). *Families and change: Coping with stressful events and transitions* (3rd Ed.), (pp. 379–401). Thousand Oaks, CA: Sage.

Google. (2016). Work-life balance. Results retrieved on 2/16/2016 from www.google.com.

Guest, D.E. (2002). Perspectives on the study of work-life balance. *Social Science Information, 41*(2), 255–279.

Hesse, A.R. (2002). Secondary trauma: How working with trauma survivors affects therapists. *Clinical Social Work Journal, 30*(3), 293–309.

Hill, E.J., Hawkins, A.J., Ferris, M., & Weitzman, M. (2001). Finding an extra day a week: The positive influence of perceived job flexibility on work and family life balance. *Family Relations, 50*(1), 49–58.

Lakey, B., & Cohen, S. (2000). Social support theory and measurement. In S. Cohen, L.G. Underwood, & B.H. Gottlieb (Eds.), *Social support measurement and intervention: A guide for health and social scientists* (pp. 29–52). Oxford: Oxford University Press.

Meichenbaum, D. (2007). Self-care for trauma psychotherapists and caregivers: Individual, social and organizational interventions. In 11th Annual Conference of the Melissa Institute for Violence Prevention and Treatment of Victims of Violence, Miami, FL. Retrieved from http://www.melissainstitute.org/documents/Meichenbaum_SelfCare_11thconf. pdf.

Nelson-Gardell, D. & Harris, D. (2003). Childhood abuse history, secondary traumatic stress, and child welfare workers. *Child Welfare, 82*(1).

Newell, J.M., & MacNeil, G.A. (2010). Professional burnout, vicarious trauma, secondary traumatic stress, and compassion fatigue. *Best Practices in Mental Health, 6*(2), 57–68.
Pearlman, L.A. & Saakvitne, K.W. (1995). Treating therapists with vicarious traumatization and secondary traumatic stress disorders. In C.R. Figley (Ed.), *Compassion fatigue: Coping with secondary traumatic stress disorder in those who treat the traumatized.* (pp. 150–177). New York, NY: Brunner/Mazel.
Phipps, A.B., & Byrne, M.K. (2003). Brief interventions for secondary trauma: Review and recommendations. *Stress and Health, 19*(3), 139–147.
Pope, K.S. & Vasquez, M.J. (2005). *How to survive and thrive as a therapist: Information, ideas, and resources for psychologists in practice.* Washington, D.C.: American Psychological Association.
Quick, J.C., Tetrick, L.E., Adkins, J., & Klunder, C. (2003). *Occupational health psychology.* New York: John Wiley & Sons.
Ray, E.B., & Miller, K.I. (1994). Social support, home/work stress, and burnout: Who can help? *The Journal of Applied Behavioral Science, 30*(3), 357–373.
Smith, J., & Gardner, D. (2007). Factors affecting employee use of work-life balance initiatives. *New Zealand Journal of Psychology, 36*(1), 3.
Stamm, H.B. (1999). *Secondary traumatic stress: Self-Care issues for clinicians, researchers, and educators.* Baltimore, MD: Sidran Press.
Taylor, S. (2006). *Clinician's guide to PTSD: A cognitive-behavioral approach.* New York, NY: Guilford Press.
Whetten, D. & Cameron, K.S. (2010). Developing managing skills, (8th Ed.). Saddle River, NJ: Prentice Hall.

SUGGESTED READING

Ashkenas, R. (2012). Forget work-life balance: It's time for work-life blend. *Forbes.* Retrieved from http://www.forbes.com/sites/ronashkenas/2012/10/19/forget-work-life-balance-its-time-for-work-life-blend/#329002cb3e2f.
American Psychological Association. (2004). The report of the APA Presidential Initiative on Work and Families: Aligning public policies, schools, and communities with the realities of contemporary families and the workplace. Washington, D.C.: Author. Retrieved from http://www.apa.org/pubs/info/reports/work-family.aspx.
Harris, B. & Sullivan, A.L. (2013). Work-life balance in academic careers. *Educational Psychology Faculty Publications.* Retrieved from http://works.bepress.com/bryn_harris/20/.
Houston, D.M. (ed.) (2005). *Work-life balance in the 21st century.* New York, NY: Palgrave Macmillan.
Loflin, J. (2015). Millennials don't want work-life balance. Retrieved from https://www.linkedin.com/pulse/millennials-dont-want-work-life-balance-jones-loflin.

McCann, I.L., & Pearlman, L.A. (1990). Vicarious traumatization: A framework for understanding the psychological effects of working with victims. *Journal of Traumatic Stress, 3*(1), 131–149.

Personal Goal Setting: Planning to Live Your Life Your Way. (n.d.). Retrieved on 7/16/2015 from http://www.mindtools.com.

Schultheiss, D.E.P. (2006). The interface of work and family life. *Professional Psychology: Research and Practice, 37*(4), 334.

Stamm, B. (1995). *Secondary traumatic stress: Self-care issues for clinicians, researchers, and educators.* Baltimore, MD: The Sidran Press.

Super's life-space theory: a useful framework for achieving balance. (n.d.) Retrieved on 7/16/2015 from http://www.calpro-online.org/eric/docs/niles/niles4.pdf.

Chapter **9**

Twenty-five Strategies for Engaging in Self-care

Laura Hensley and Andrea Schultz-Duncan

As mental health providers, we are very familiar with the concepts of boundaries and setting limits. We talk about these issues with our clients and colleagues, and ideally practice setting limits and boundaries in our own everyday lives. The purpose of this chapter is to identify some common self-care strategies, and to discuss why they are needed and how to implement them.

Within the private practice setting, we face a number of challenges that are not necessarily present in other areas of our field. While we have the benefit of often being able to set our own hours, we are largely responsible for making sure that we are taking appropriate care of our clients. Financial safety nets are only available when we have set them up for ourselves. There are no "backup" plans. Emergency coverage often falls on us (unless there is some other predetermined plan), and we are often isolated (whether by virtue of setting up an individual practice or being in a group practice where others largely keep to themselves). These factors can create quite a challenge, especially when we get sick or simply need a break! Self-care is important for all clinicians. Without making sure that we are in the best possible frame of mind to help others, there is no possible way that we can maintain our effectiveness. In this chapter, we present 25 concrete strategies for taking care of yourself in a private practice setting.

1. BALANCE PROFESSIONAL LIFE AND PERSONAL LIFE

As a group, mental health professionals tend to be empathic and giving of time. While necessary in this line of work, if you do not balance the demands of your professional commitments with those of your personal commitments, you run the risk of burnout, exhaustion, and damage to relationships. Striking a balance between professional and personal life can be particularly difficult. Not only do personal differences come into play in this situation, ethical responsibilities, financial needs, organizational demands, and personal commitments are sometimes at odds. Additionally, if working in an independent practice or in a practice that lacks a sense of group cohesion among providers, maintaining the necessary awareness of this balance may be a challenge.

The balance may look different from one week to the next, but awareness of personal and professional priorities is very important in being able to achieve an overall balance. Some basic guidelines may help to at least start the process. Keep work from creeping into your personal life as much as possible. This may require "unplugging" from time to time. Setting limits around checking voicemails and emails, and identifying a time of the day when you stop working until the next day, are simple strategies that can be employed to achieve this goal. Informing and explaining this boundary to clients, students, and colleagues may not only help them to respect the boundaries you set, but may model healthy boundaries that they may also benefit from setting. It is also important to consider these strategies as a means of protecting your time at home. By ensuring that work tasks are completed during work hours, you can limit the amount of time that you are spending at home playing catch-up. It is also important to consider the times that we do "a small favor" for a client. These favors tend to add up, taking away from the time that we are completing necessary tasks and limiting our ability to maintain this professional/personal balance. At times, we may need to develop new policies and procedures that more clearly define what we will and will not do for clients. For example, you might state that when writing a letter or completing paperwork at the request of the client, a charge will be incurred if the completion of the task is done outside of session time, or if it takes more than 15 minutes. This is of course something that needs to be determined by the specific needs of the client as well as the demands of the clinician; however, consciously thinking about such strategies can prevent future problems.

2. PACE OF THE DAY

As an extension of the importance of balance between personal and professional life, it is also important to recognize that the pace of your work day can be an important aspect of self-care. If you have clients scheduled back-to-back from 8 AM until 6 PM with 30 minutes to write notes, return phone calls, respond to emails, and eat something (probably a handful of popcorn or a spoonful of peanut butter), and if you can only take a bathroom break when clients come late, are you going to be very effective therapeutically? We all have demands that make us feel compelled to see as many clients as possible. Financial demands, productivity demands, and the clinical needs of our caseloads can all result in significant pressure to perhaps take on more than we can reasonably be expected to manage.

The control that you may or may not have over your time may be limited by the organization where you work or the population that you work with in your setting. Control over our schedules must often be balanced with revenue production. Here are some guidelines that may help to start the process of fixing this very common problem. When you take breaks, schedule separate times when you can work on administrative tasks versus times that you can sit and collect your thoughts, use relaxation or mindfulness techniques, and eat something nutritious. Speaking to others about the boundaries that you want to set may be helpful in identifying strategies for meeting expectations as well as maintaining mental health and physical well-being. In many private practice settings, clinicians have significant say over when and how much they need to work; however, as you know, we all still have to consider the impact that this may or may not have on income. Identifying your needs is a helpful first step. Consider the time needed between clients, how often a longer break may be necessary, the number of clients that you may need to see to feel financially comfortable, and what your personal schedule requires. Once you have identified these needs, you can then start working backwards to finalize the schedule that works best for you.

3. KEEP UP WITH NEW INFORMATION

The mental health field is ever changing and growing. New research is being done all the time which may have implications for how we treat and interact with our clients. It is hard to keep up with all of this new information that is being generated, and with a full caseload, the time available to read all of this information is just not available.

The name of the game is "divide and conquer." Take the time to consult with colleagues and discuss recent trainings attended, share information about books and articles you have read, and take advantage of supervision opportunities. Practices with multiple providers may offer opportunities to meet, and this may also be available through local professional organizations. Accepting invitations to teach classes or seminars can be another way of achieving this goal. Those working in private practice often do not have access to online databases without paying significant amounts of money. Gaining access to this type of resource through academic institutions (if you want to teach), joining listservs relevant to your work, or sharing the cost of journal subscriptions or databases with other providers can make keeping up with research easier and more affordable.

4. IDENTIFY AND DEAL WITH "HOT BUTTONS"

While many of us like to think we are free of bias, we are not. We all have things that come up in our work that might be triggers, baggage from previous experiences, or "hot buttons." Personal values and experiences may influence these buttons. Some buttons are likely to be more active than others and therefore may be more or less of a problem. Anyone can push these buttons, but from a professional standpoint, when colleagues and clients push these buttons, it can influence the quality and direction of these relationships.

Awareness is the first part of the solution. Becoming aware of and understanding these buttons allows us to more readily address and solve the problem. Solutions and outcomes may vary. Through professional consultations, one may be able to develop a reframed understanding of the situation, which improves one's ability to respond professionally. One may need to reasonably limit one's practice if necessary. At times, individual therapy may be helpful to learn how to let go of negative energy picked up in session, set emotional boundaries around the difficult things that we hear, and identify useful methods to let go of stress.

5. PRACTICE WHAT YOU PREACH!

In our clinical practice, we help clients look at the world in a new way; we allow them to challenge their negative beliefs and encourage them to do great things. Sometimes we find ourselves struggling with the same difficulties that our clients do; feeling overwhelmed with sadness or anxiety, struggling to feel like things could get better. Maybe we're in a new situation, adjusting to change, or over-stressed. Maybe we have allowed ourselves to become overwhelmed or burned out. Whatever the reason, the skills we use with clients can be helpful in getting through our own struggles.

If you find yourself feeling overwhelmed, check in; ask, "What am I doing to take care of myself? How's my sleep? Am I being active? How much alcohol am I consuming? Am I eating balanced healthy meals?"

When we are overwhelmed, we can minimize vulnerability to negative emotions by using the same skills that we teach our clients. If you notice negative emotions, don't assume your perception is accurate. Talking with others to identify your negative thoughts can be effective in challenging your distortions and gaining a new, healthier perspective. Just like with our clients, if we allow ourselves to become overwhelmed by negative distortions, we will be negatively affected.

6. SAY "NO"

As helpers we often find ourselves over-committed. Seeing others in need, whether it be clients, coworkers, or people in the community, can draw out our empathic side. While this is an incredible gift and betterment for the communities and people we are near, it can be overwhelming and draining when we commit ourselves too much. We've already mentioned striking a balance between work and personal lives. Now we are addressing a deeper issue. Allowing a break from the constant doing for others and emotional drain that often accompanies that is an important step in self-care.

Saying no to requests can be a difficult task. However, prioritizing the events and relationships that are most important to you is essential to your own ability to feel content. There is simply not enough time to accept all requests and invitations. Saying no to requests is not just reserved for times when you are already committed. Making time for leisure, relaxing, and simply wasting time is also important. Think about the most enjoyable days or weeks in your life and try to model your days and weeks from that. How much time in your most enjoyable days was spent relaxing? With family? With friends? Completing obligations? Keep that balance in mind as you commit yourself to future engagements. Will this new event or obligation subtract from the things you most enjoy? Allow yourself time to consider requests before committing. At times the pressure we feel to please others can make an idea seem good, and it is not until later that we feel the regret or overwhelmed state when we recognize how this new obligation fits with what we have already taken on. Remind yourself that you cannot do everything, especially when you are not making time for the things that reenergize you the most.

7. PRACTICE MINDFULNESS

The culture we live in is fast-paced, competitive, and often chaotic. Multitasking is viewed as a skill to develop and highlight on resumes. Pressure to do more, offer more, and be the best is often demanded in practice. However, the pressure to constantly do more can become overwhelming. Mistakes are made, we are over scheduled, and we find ourselves missing out on the important things because we are not able to turn off our minds to enjoy them.

Mindfulness is a purposeful step away from that culture. It is a slowing down of your body and mind, and being more attuned to yourself. The simplest way to begin mindfulness is through your breathing. Set aside 5 minutes to focus on your breathing and nothing else. Start by simply tuning into the breaths you are taking. Notice the way your lungs expand as you fill them with air. Continue to fill your lungs with air until you are completely full, then push all of the air out using your stomach. Slow your breaths down, taking 3 to 5 seconds to inhale through your nose and 5 to 7 seconds to exhale through your mouth. The addition of progressive muscle relaxation can aid in increasing your focus in the moment and in reducing stress levels. Progressive muscle relaxation is the pairing of deep breathing with the purposeful tightening and releasing of individual muscles or muscle groups. Engaging in a more formal practice of meditation or yoga can also help you to calm and focus your mind.

More information about diaphragmatic breathing and a script for progressive muscle relaxation can be found in *The Anxiety and Phobia Workbook* (Bourne, 2005).

Resources for meditation can be found in *Mindfulness in Clinical Practice* (Sears, Tirch, & Denton, 2011).

8. EAT WELL

Sometimes there are just not enough hours in the day. If you have a full caseload and limited time to catch up on therapy notes or other administrative tasks, something has to drop to the bottom of the to-do list. For many people, eating something nutritious may be that task. When we consider the mental and physical benefits of healthy eating, the struggle is how to make sure that this is something that we can do for ourselves during the work day.

Part of the solution may involve doing meal or food preparation ahead of time. For example, keep some healthy food options in the office. Bring precut vegetables from home, keep a bag of mixed nuts in your desk drawer, or bring preportioned leftovers from the delicious dinner you made over the weekend in the break room. Ideally, schedule time specifically for eating instead of eating, phone calls, emails, letter/report writing, etc. Following general guidelines about maintaining balanced nutrition and eating things that "come from the ground," but also letting yourself indulge from time to time, make eating more healthy, enjoyable, and sustainable. For more information about eating well, see Nutrition.gov (http://www.nutrition.gov/).

9. SLEEP

Working long hours and balancing social and family needs often results in time being taken away from sleep. Some nights, even when we allot the time to sleep, we find ourselves lying in bed wide awake. We know the importance of sleep; we talk to clients about it all the time. Yet somehow when it comes to our own sleep pattern, we find ourselves missing out. Difficulty focusing, careless mistakes, and irritability often accompany a lack of sleep. We need to make sleep a priority.

Basic sleep hygiene is essential to being effective clinicians. Most adults need between 7 and 9 hours of sleep every night. As appealing as the snooze button can seem, maintaining a daily bedtime and wake-up time helps to keep our circadian rhythm in sync. For those of us struggling to fall asleep even when we make the time, we need to ensure that when it is time to sleep our mind and body are ready. Creating a bedtime routine that allows for relaxation and calming of your body and mind can help prepare your body for sleep. Part of that bedtime routine should include the elimination of bright lights, including those from screens on television, computers, cell phones, and tablets, at least 1 hour prior to your scheduled bedtime. Elimination of caffeine from your diet after 2 PM is another way to help calm your body and mind for bed. The environment you sleep in can have a great deal of impact as well. Creating a calm environment to sleep can be important; make sure you have a comfortable bed and a clutter-free room to rest your mind. Keep your room as dark and cool as possible, ideally between 60 and 67 degrees, to promote restful sleep. If you notice your mind has trouble calming down at night, try keeping a small tablet beside your bed to jot down worries, thoughts, and insights as they come. Writing them down can help you to turn your mind off and relax rather than ruminating in bed or worrying you will forget to take care of it when you wake. With these small steps you can give sleep the place of priority it needs in your life.

10. PROCESS YOUR THOUGHTS AND FEELINGS

One of the best parts of being in private practice is having a network of strong colleagues that you can rely on for consultation and client referrals. One of the downsides is that all of those wonderful clinicians are now your friends. Going to people that we consider friends for clinical health feels impossible, and can be ethically complicated. What happens when you have a crisis? What ways can you process your own thoughts and feelings when needed? Ongoing support in the helping field is a necessity. We are taking on the stresses and burdens of other people, which can eat away at our own mental health. In addition to the emotional toll of our profession, we are also human; meaning we are susceptible to the same mental health concerns as every other person.

Personal reflection through journaling or daily meditation can be a helpful way to reduce our own distress. Journaling and guided readings allow us the ability to reflect on our own perception and events in our lives. Consulting with peers can allow perspective and help in emotionally coping with the stress of difficult clients. If you are lucky enough to work in a larger practice, this type of consultation can occur daily. For those of us in smaller practices, we must seek out peer consultation through groups and planned events with colleagues. Finding a personal therapist outside of your network of friends is an important part of ongoing mental health care for yourself. This gives you a safe space to be the helped, instead of the helper. Many successful clinicians find themselves coming in and out of therapy throughout their careers for the same reason that our high-functioning clients do; because, none of us can really do this alone.

11. BE PHYSICALLY ACTIVE

Your body was made to move. Movement, whether it be exercise, hunting, gardening, chores, walking, or yoga, is essential to your body's health and your mental well-being. You, however, have a job where the majority of your day is spent sitting in a chair talking to others, sitting in a chair writing notes, sitting in a chair making phone calls, and quite possibly going home to sit in a chair to watch TV. While the job you have is fulfilling in so many ways, it is not fulfilling the need for movement that your body has.

How can you integrate movement into your daily routine? Of course joining a gym or going for a daily run would be ideal, but what if you aren't motivated to do that? What if you don't have the time to commit to an hour of exercise? How can we increase physical activity other ways? Think about the activities of your day, and identify ways to increase movement in what you are already doing. Stand while making phone calls, while doing chores, or even relaxing at home. Find fun activities to become involved in at least once or twice a week, such as a dance class, kayaking, or even rollerblading. Connecting with other active people can help you be inspired to be more active as well.

12. SCHEDULE TIME "OFF-CALL"

We all know the importance of being available for our clients, at any time, to ensure that they are not in an emergency situation alone. Think about the significance of being on call for your clients, any moment of the day, every day of the week, and every week of the year. Being on call often means that your life has to be structured around the possibility that a crisis could happen at any moment. Carrying your phone to church, weddings, and graduations. Walking out of movies to take a call, interrupting an intimate moment to make sure it's not a client trying to get a hold of you. The reality of being on call every moment means that you are not able to destress in a real way. You are not able to turn off the professional side completely because you know it could be turned back on at a moment's notice.

Effectively sharing on call responsibilities with other people in your practice is a huge help in reducing this burden. Having an on-call rotation that each clinician takes only once every few weeks is an option many practices use. Other practices coordinate weeks off-call by covering the on-call responsibilities for each other's caseloads a few times a year. Many clinicians take crisis calls while out of town, or on vacation. But just because you can answer your phone, doesn't mean it's a good idea to always do that. Coordinating time with a colleague to cover each other's on-call crises can be a simple way to allow yourself a break and to really relax. What if you are in practice alone, does that make taking time off call any less important? Of course not. While you want to ensure that confidentiality is maintained, having clients sign an agreement for a colleague at another practice to be involved in their critical care can be an easy way to give yourself a break. Coverage could be arranged by forwarding calls; however, it can be done more simply and will minimize confidentiality concerns if you simply give clients a secondary crisis number to call on weeks in which you will not be available. By giving clients a secondary number to call, they are fully informed that they are calling a clinician outside of your practice. Both you and your clients can relax knowing this is a professional that you trust to take care of your client's concerns while you are taking care of yourself. Explanations of confidentiality and HIPAA compliance related to outside persons covering on-call can be found through HIPAA's website (www.hhs.gov).

13. GO ON A HOMETOWN ADVENTURE

We all love going on vacation; the new sites, foods, the relaxation of being stress free, responsibility free. Sometimes though, schedules or budget don't allow us to take a trip out of town. This doesn't mean that we have to stay confined to our office working 365 days a year. What is it that you love about taking vacation? Is it trying new food, exploring new areas, experiencing a new culture, going on an outdoor adventure?

Many of the parts you love about vacation can be found right in your own backyard. No matter where you live there are restaurants within an hour that you haven't tried. During our regular lives we don't always try new restaurants. We often go to the same restaurants and even eat the same thing; having variety is part of what makes vacations so exciting. Taking a meal vacation is a simple, affordable way to have some of the vacation experience. Find a restaurant that you've never been to and order a meal that you've never had. Maybe try an outdoor adventure that you love. Learn more about places to hike, athletic courses you can run, and rivers or lakes you can kayak near your hometown. Many of us take the culture of our hometown for granted. Whether you live in a big city or small rural community, there are cultural pieces unique to your town. Travel and city or county websites can be a great resource to help you see your community with fresh eyes like a tourist does. The sites may have information about cultural events, local landmarks, and activities that are available to you. Maybe there is a museum you haven't visited since you were a child, or an updated exhibit that you didn't realize had changed. You can find information about local festivals, concerts, or natural wonders near your home that can give you the same excitement that you would have as a tourist. If lying on the beach is one of the best parts of vacation for you, find a way to make your own beach by going to a local pool, lake, or river. You don't have to be on the coast to be at the beach; recreate the pieces that you love best and experience them even if for just an afternoon.

14. BE ADVENTUROUS

There is nothing like getting stuck in a rut to make us feel unfulfilled. While the solution seems easy, sometimes it is hard to motivate yourself to break out of it. Whether the lack of motivation comes from being comfortable, lack of awareness of what new opportunities are available to you, fear of the outcomes, or perhaps feeling that you don't have the time (or energy) to get out of your comfort zone, trying something new has the potential for increasing a sense of accomplishment.

Before you can try something new, you have to research what new experiences are available in your area, such as new foods/restaurants, sports, organizations, or classes. While these new experiences could be related to your work, sometimes it is better to get out of "work mode" and do something completely out of the ordinary. Local news websites, city-specific resources (online or in print), or the many coupon websites that are available (e.g. Groupon, Living Social, Amazon Local, etc.) are all good resources. Another helpful factor may be finding someone that is willing to seek out new experiences by your side. Whether this be a significant other, friend, sibling, parent, or other family member, this may serve as an opportunity to strengthen relationships and develop shared experiences to talk about in the future.

15. RECONNECT WITH YOUR 20-YEAR-OLD SELF (I.E., WHO YOU WERE BEFORE YOU BECAME A "PROFESSIONAL")

This is a tricky problem. So many people in the mental health profession are trained to feel as though they need to maintain some level of professionalism, even when they are not engaged in professional activities, in the event that they run into a client/former client or the family member of a client. For those who have experienced this, it can be an awkward encounter made more awkward if they are unable, for whatever reason, to put on that professional hat immediately. For example, if you are in a situation where your child is having a meltdown in the middle of a grocery store, where you are out in some sort of outfit that you would NEVER wear in your office (even if the situation calls for it), or simply having a glass of wine or a beer at your favorite restaurant, an already awkward situation can become worse. So the question is, how do you maintain a connection with your nonprofessional self or the person you were before you took on that professional persona?

Not that you necessarily want to revisit the days of your youth when you may have stayed up all night, lounged all day, and then did it all over again, but you do have to be realistic about your expectations for leisure time. Enjoying the things that you have always enjoyed keeps you from feeling that your job has taken over, and therefore reduces the risk of burnout. You can still take part in various activities that might not be strictly considered "professional" without getting out of control. Sometimes teaching balance means that you have to model that for your clients, and might include doing something silly like participating in a locally held cultural event which requires dressing in costume or participating in local festivals and events. In certain situations, having a conversation with clients about how you handle situations in a public setting and expressly telling them that you are a person and do exist outside of the office can help to prevent any awkwardness and allow you to enjoy life more.

16. DO SOMETHING YOU ENJOY EVERYDAY

Especially with a new practice, but even for those of us who has been in practice for a very long time, we devote a huge amount of time to our clients, our professional development, and trying to run a business. While most of us truly enjoy the work we do, our work cannot be our whole self. Outside of being a mental health professional, what do you enjoy doing? When was the last time that you remember doing the things that you enjoy? Not taking care of others, not doing something because you have to, or out of obligation, but because you truly enjoyed it?

Effective self-care involves daily reminders of the things you love; spending time doing things that bring you joy. It's not realistic to think that you can devote hours every day just doing things for fun. It's also not realistic to think that you don't have any time in your day to do something fun. Enjoyable activities can take just a few minutes on a busy day and can take an entire weekend when you have time to spare. While some people enjoy hobbies, others enjoy sports. Some people enjoy listening to music, while others enjoy watching a movie. For some people, spending time with children or animals can bring peace, while for others a loud concert or busy social scene brings them joy. Finding time to curl up with a good book, catching up with an old friend, pampering yourself with a massage or yoga class, or training for the upcoming marathon; whatever brings you joy simply by doing it, needs a place in your day, every day. Consider what is stopping you from including these things in your day already. Can you find time to devote to bringing more joy to your life? Imagine the change made possible by simply adding a few minutes of joy.

17. TIME WITH FRIENDS AND FAMILY

Sometimes by the end of the day or over the weekend, we just don't have the time or energy to do it all. Whether that is keeping up with laundry, doing yard work, spending time with our significant other/children (human or animal), or making time for friends, there are only so many hours in the day. Fitting everything in that needs to be done sometimes feels like an impossible feat, and few of those tasks feel like they can wait for another day.

The solution to this particular problem is likely to look very different for different people. For some, enlisting or offering help with certain tasks, scheduling time to spend with people that you haven't seen in a while, or changing your priorities are all possible ways of solving this problem. The goal is to spend time with people that make you feel good. Maybe this is planning a grocery shopping trip with a friend or scheduling a potluck dinner with family and friends. Finding ways of being more productive or delegating tasks (e.g., putting your spouse and kids to work) may decrease the time spent doing these "necessary" tasks and free up time for leisure. Maintaining a relationship with your colleagues is also really important. Spending time together outside of work and taking time to have lunch together can provide an opportunity to give and receive support from others that have similar experiences and points of view in terms of professional outlook.

18. SCHEDULE DATE NIGHT

As an extension to the problem associated with finding time to spend with friends and family, there are certain relationships that you want to and should foster more. While many people think of a “date night” as being focused on a significant other or romantic partner, you can also schedule a date night with a best friend, child, sibling, or anyone else with whom you have a significant relationship. The biggest problem with this is that again, there are just not enough hours in the day. Maybe there are obstacles such as work schedules to take into account, or the need for child care or financial constraints that limit our abilities to schedule this time; however, it is necessary to maintain these very close relationships.

Again, it is important to consider your resources. If you have friends with children, set up a schedule where the children go to one house and you and your significant other can go on a date. Find activities in your area that are free or low cost, such as farmer’s markets, festivals, concerts, volunteer organizations, etc. You can also set aside time at the end of the day, so you and an important person can talk on the phone, play a game, or watch a movie together to allow for some quality time. Physical intimacy may also be an important part of these relationships. Giving and receiving various levels of appropriate physical affection can be an important component of this dedicated time.

19. GET YOUR STUFF TOGETHER!

When things get hectic, even the most well planned organizational system can fall to pieces. While people tend to be more or less overtly sensitive to clutter and disorganization, chaos can make many people feel scattered and uncomfortable. It can also make doing what we need to do, personally and professionally, more difficult, time consuming, or even more expensive. For example, you meet a new client, and know that 5 months ago you made the most perfect handout for the problem that they are reporting, but you have NO idea where you put it. Maybe you have a project you are working on at home and you know you bought something a year ago that you can use to complete the project, but you can’t find it. You may have to remake that handout or go to the store to buy the same thing again, hoping that the store still carries the item.

As we all know, developing and maintaining an organizational system can be time consuming. Sometimes we need help figuring out the best method for this, and other times it seems to be a relatively easy fix. Setting timelines for going through things, eliminating items that do not need to be retained, identifying things that you need to keep handy, and donating usable items (that you no longer need) can all be helpful strategies. For some, the task of developing an organizational system is overwhelming, and it might be worth finding a friend or family member or even hiring a professional organizer to help out. For tips about organization, look at home-based websites like HGTV, Real Simple, Pinterest, and search "organization." For more information about finding a professional organizer, see the National Association of Professional Organizers (http://www.napo.net/).

20. SET GOALS

We often work with clients on setting goals. Goals provide a framework and direction for self-improvement, and help provide motivation for positive changes. This is something that everyone can benefit from. For some, this may be a very structured endeavor, but for others, there may be more fluidity to these goals. The point is to set short- and long-term goals for both personal and professional domains.

Identifying areas of improvement is typically the first step. Identifying things not only professionally but personally that might make your life easier or more fulfilling can lead to great things! Maybe you want to brush up on that guitar you have been moving from place to place for the last 15 years, delve into a new professional interest so you can expand your practice, or simply find time to do 10 minutes of stretching every day. Any one of these changes may improve some aspect of your life and help to create the balance for which we all strive.

21. RECONNECT WITH NATURE

Most of us spend our days behind walls, doors, windows, and steel. Sunshine is felt through pane glass, and fresh air is filtered through ventilation. Between the time when commuting to and from work and the time we spend at our office, the majority of our lives are spent away from nature. When was the last time that you were outside for longer than 5 minutes? How often do you make time to watch the sunset, gaze at the stars, or explore the outdoors? What do you think you miss out on by locking yourself away inside? What could you gain by connecting with nature?

Making time for nature is a purposeful way to relax your body and mind. Whether you find time to go on a short walk during lunch, or a grand excursion on your days off, this reconnecting to nature can allow you to gain perspective and mindfulness. Regardless of where you live, there are opportunities to spend more time in nature. Look into local parks and protected grounds to find trails, creeks, and mountains to climb. If hiking does not appeal to you, making time to watch the clouds while you picnic, or looking for birds in your neighborhood may be an alternative more your style. Whether you are in a park, in the city, or your own neighborhood, the simple step of taking time to notice the beauty of nature through flowers, trees, and wildlife can bring relaxation. Go find your fresh air.

22. LEARN A NEW SKILL

As children we were always learning. Learning how to walk, how to read, how to ride a bike. As adults, we frequently limit our learning to areas where we are already comfortable; we learn more about our field of study, we learn more about daily living skills. Somehow as adults we either forget to make time to master new skills, or we fail to realize the significance of getting the sense of joy after reaching that next milestone. We've talked about the importance of trying new things; mastering a skill is taking that to the next level.

It's more than getting out of your comfort zone. Learning a new skill is allowing yourself to see real progress in your ability. Imagine if you started learning a new language—it would be easy to see yourself progress as your vocabulary increases, or as you begin understanding conversations in that language. If you took up music, you would see your skills progress as you work on more and more challenging pieces. If you took up art, you would see your progress as your work becomes more skilled and beautiful. It is with the milestones of progress that learning a new skill takes you from experiencing joy doing something you like, to feeling pride in yourself.

23. CONTRIBUTE TO OTHERS

Our work lives are filled with contributions to others; we provide stability and consistency for the clients we see. Our job is one that is filled with opportunities to improve our communities. At times though, we are reminded that we are also doing our jobs because we need to. We have bills to pay and households to support. In some way we are aware of that driving force, as a part of why we contribute to our clients in the ways we do.

Contributing is about more than that. Finding groups and individuals to give back to, with no expectation of payment, allows us to focus on the giving, and can help alleviate feelings of stress or discontent in our own lives. Contributing can be done in small simple ways, like buying the food for the car behind you at the drive through, or making a donation to an organization you care about. You can use your skill set in your contributions, like taking on a pro bono client, or volunteering with the Red Cross Disaster Relief teams as a mental health volunteer. You can contribute through your religious organization, or you can find opportunities to volunteer by contacting local nonprofits or looking at a national database like the United Way. Volunteer opportunities can be commitments of a few hours one afternoon, or be ongoing commitments to help with the organization you are passionate about. Whether big or small, your contributions make a difference to your community, and within yourself.

24. EXPRESS GRATITUDE

Life can be so stressful and busy. There are days where it seems nothing is working out, almost as though the universe is working against us. Not surprisingly, we notice the things in life that we focus our attention on; and those things can seem to multiply.

In the same way that focusing on negative aspects of life can draw our attention to other negative things, focusing on the positive things in life has the same ability to draw our attention to more positive things. Making time to express gratitude to others for the things they do in our lives helps us to bring our attention to the supportive people we have. Thanking a police officer or community worker that you pass helps you to notice the people in your city that are working to improve your life and keep you safe. Expressing appreciation to everyone who helps you during the day draws your attention to the small details that are making your day easier. It also allows you to maintain perspective on the things that don't work out as planned because they are within the context of otherwise positive experiences. Setting aside time each day to think about or write down the things that you are grateful for is another way to turn your focus to the positive. You can think of both the things that others did for you, as well as things that just happened, such as getting home just before a rainstorm, snagging a front row parking spot, or making the perfect cup of tea. Keeping this sense of gratitude in the forefront of your mind is a powerful way to encourage a positive mood.

25. SELF-CARE—JUST DO IT

As with many of these areas, finding time is an ever present battle. As mental health professionals, we preach the importance of self-care, but sometimes we are really bad about taking our own advice. So the question remains, how do you make time for something that often ends up falling to the bottom of the to-do list?

While this is easier said than done, you must make self-care a priority. Remember all those little things you tell your clients in an effort to be helpful. You can't take care of someone else if you don't take care of yourself. If you are expecting yourself to be a "Super Clinician," able to give and give but always having a ready supply of more, you are going to fail. Engaging in regular self-care can help us clinically by identifying strategies or problem solving pitfalls. This is wisdom that we can pass on to our clients, allowing us to honestly and genuinely encourage our clients to prioritize self-care.

The intention of this chapter is not to shame you or make you feel bad about your self-care. We do not expect perfection. We do not expect you to implement all of these strategies in the next month. The hope is that you can find one or two strategies or new ideas for how to improve your work and home life that you can start working on, making them your own. While many of these ideas and examples have originated from our own experiences, they are certainly not the only ways of implementing change. Feel free to borrow and come up with your own strategies as you see fit.

For more general information about self-care and boundary setting within the mental health field, see the American Psychological Association (www.apa.org), the American Mental Health Counselors Association (http://www.amhca.org), the National Association for Social Workers (http://www.naswdc.org), the American Counseling Association (http://www.counseling.org), and other national and local professional organizations.

REFERENCES

Bourne, E.J. (2005). *The anxiety and phobia workbook.* (6th Ed.). Oakland, CA: New Harbinger Publications.

Sears, R.W., Tirch, D.D., & Denton, R.B. (2011). *Mindfulness in clinical practice.* Sarasota, FL: Professional Resource Exchange.

Index

For Product Safety Concerns and Information please contact our EU
representative GPSR@taylorandfrancis.com
Taylor & Francis Verlag GmbH, Kaufingerstraße 24, 80331 München, Germany

www.ingramcontent.com/pod-product-compliance
Ingram Content Group UK Ltd.
Pitfield, Milton Keynes, MK11 3LW, UK
UKHW022202190926
475702UK00003B/168

* 9 7 8 1 1 3 8 9 3 5 8 8 4 *